Bikram Yoga

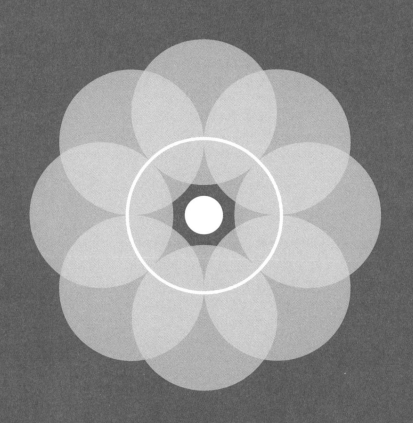

Bikram Yoga

The Guru Behind
Hot Yoga Shows the Way
to Radiant Health
and Personal Fulfillment

Bikram Choudhury

WM
WILLIAM MORROW
An Imprint of *HarperCollins*Publishers

This book is intended to be informational and should not be considered a substitute for advice from a medical professional, whom the reader should consult before beginning any diet or exercise regimen, and before taking any dietary supplements or other medications. The author and publisher expressly disclaim responsibility for any adverse effects arising from the use or application of the information contained in this book.

HarperCollins books may be purchased for educational, business, or sales promotional use. For information please write: Special Markets Department, HarperCollins Publishers, 10 East 53rd Street, New York, NY 10022.

Designed by Lovedog Studio

Photographs: page 105, 114, 124, 150, 161, 168, 172, 178, 188, 193, 199, 200, 203, 206 by Bisu Ghosh; 14, 27, 100, 109, 118, 127, 131, 136, 139, 143, 146, 157, 175, 185, 196 by Stephen Danelian.

Library of Congress Cataloging-in-Publication Data
978-0-060-56808-5
ISBN-10: 0-06-056808-9

13 14   ❖ / COU   20 19 18 17 16 15 14 13 12 11

This book is dedicated to my late father Kali Kinkar Choudhury, and my late older brothers, Ashim ("George") and Asis.

And to my wife and children: Rajashree, Laju, and Anurag. Good things come in small packages and my immediate family is the world to me.

I wish to thank these people for their help in the creation of this book:

John Burnham—With one phone call, he made the whole thing possible.

Elizabeth Leanse—She stuck with me, never giving up on me, and that's ultimately why this book is being published. All my love and thanks—I can't wait to do the next one with you!

Kris Dahl—My agent, she was the trusted guide who led me and Rajashree through the world of publishing, and this book is the result.

Craig Villani—Everybody knows I'm not a writer, I'm a speaker. Craig, with his incredible understanding of my yoga—not just the technical, teaching parts but also the emotions behind them—created this book.

John Capouya—He was the editor we needed, and when we needed him most, he appeared.

Anne-Marie Bennstrom—After my beloved guru, Bishnu Charan Ghosh, left us, she came along and took over the steering wheel on my spiritual journey. And I'm very happy and grateful to say that she really knows how to drive.

Contents

Part Three:
Living Yoga

Warning:
"I Will Tell You the Truth"

IN INDIA, WE HAVE A HINDI SAYING: *Satch, Bohot, Karwa, Hi.*
Roughly translated it means the truth is extremely bitter like
quinine, the medicine. It is one of the hardest things in life to
swallow and digest. But like quinine we swallow it because we
know it's good for us.

This book will change your life. It might even save it. But first,
I'm going to tell you some things you may not like. I'm not going
to tell you what you want to hear, I'm going to tell you what you
need to hear. I'm going to tell you the truth.

What is this bitter truth I am asking you to swallow? That
America, my adopted country that I love so much, is facing a terrible crisis. In the history of global civilization, this is the greatest
country that ever existed. During the last 200 years, you have

built the best educational system, the best medical and scientific communities, the most impressive economy, and have created more advances in technology than any other modern society. So wouldn't it be logical to assume that here you would also have the best life in the world?

Instead I see far too many problems, and I hear too much unhappiness. Statistically the United States makes up only about 5 percent of the world's population, but its people seem to complain more than the rest of the world combined! How can this be? In this land of so much wealth and opportunity you are suffering needlessly from societal problems such as crime and a high divorce rate, and despite living in the most medically advanced nation on earth, many of you are sick and unhealthy. Here you suffer the diseases of affluence, of having *too much* food and *too many* bad choices available to you. Obesity, diabetes, arthritis, heart disease—you name it, it's a sad fact of American life.

But these physical problems are a symptom of a bigger crisis, a mental and Spiritual one. From what I see, Americans' biggest problem today can be summed up in three little words: You're not happy. Think about it: How many truly happy people do you know? Does your life give you true satisfaction, are you really content? Here in the West, and especially in the United States, you have so much, but as many of you have found, that's not where your satisfaction lies. You're lost: Now that you have everything, it feels as though you have nothing. The combined wealth, beauty, and success of the entire world cannot give you the peace you seek—and that you deserve.

Let me help you. In my country, India, we have devised a system that allows us to find happiness, even with all our poverty and material problems. Long ago we came to realize that just building a beautiful country where people can lead comfortable lives doesn't lead to lasting happiness. Before the birth of the modern West, India played at the game of materialism and was the richest country in the world for thousands of years. We realized through our failure that basing our society on achievement and wealth didn't work, and we gave it up. Instead we made our priorities humanity, Spiritualism, and love, and we seek to promote the continued evolution of all human life. To us the ultimate destination of human life is mental happiness and peace through the realization of love.

What is this system we use to take us on that journey? It's called yoga, and that's what I'm offering you in the pages of this book. Yoga can not only save your life; it will help you to save your soul. So, as you are beginning to realize, this is not just an "exercise book." Not at all, my friend, not even close.

You see, practicing Hatha Yoga—the kind my guru taught me and that I want to pass on to you—will not just prevent and treat many diseases, it also eases the mental and emotional malaise that afflicts people in the West. Yoga can give you physical health like you've never even imagined, plus a true understanding of life, including the purpose you are meant to fulfill here on Earth. Yoga is not a religion, but it is Spiritualism, the way that will help you to reach your true, unlimited potential as a human being. It helps provide answers to ultimate questions, like: "Who am I?" "Why am I here?" "What should I do with my life?"

You deserve better information and you deserve a better life. Bringing yoga to you here in America is my job, the Karmic duty I was charged with by my guru back in India. I've been teaching and practicing yoga for more than fifty years now and I've changed hundreds of thousands of lives for the better. But I can't help you if you won't face the truth and admit that you need to change. Some of you don't realize or won't admit that any problem exists—and if that's the case, how are you going to solve it?

Only after you acknowledge that you just might not have all the answers can you begin to find solutions. Admit you are going in the wrong direction, and then you can make a U-turn. Then you'll be able to save your marriage from divorce, your body and mind from drugs, your heart from lies, and your neighborhood and community from crime. Maybe none of us alone can save the world, but if each of us took the time to solve our individual problems, the world would be like heaven. At the very least, we can leave our children a better world in which to live.

Through yoga I will help you to discover that you actually *do* have the answers inside of you already—you just don't know where or how to look. I've written this book to help you see things as they truly are and not remain trapped in illusion, the tricks of the mind that we think are reality. You have been asleep for too long; it is time to wake up.

Along the way I'm going to tell you more bitter truths, and I'll be tougher on you than anything or anybody most Americans have ever experienced. Even if I wanted to write a book of lies, telling you how wonderful your life is and how the world is filled with perfect human beings, I couldn't do it. I wouldn't be able to digest the food I'd buy with the money you paid for this book.

I think you can handle the truth. Besides, speaking unpleasant but necessary truths is part of who I am, and there's no way I'm going to change now. Fire's got to burn, ice has to cool, and Bikram's got to be Bikram. I've got balls and I've got guts, so I say and do the things I think my students need, whether or not it hurts their feelings. But along with all my yelling and rough talk, my students can see the love and compassion I have for them as well. They can feel that they're healing. And I know that you will, too, because my Bikram Yoga students look better, feel better and lead happier, more fulfilling lives.

Maybe you are unwilling to listen to the truth, but that is not my problem. My responsibility rests in telling you the truth as I see it, and nothing more. So open your mind, open your heart, and listen to what I have to say. You might disagree, you might deny, but you must listen. Read this whole book before you make up your mind about me and about yoga. Come take a class at one of my studios, too. If you do these things, if you take my advice and you practice Bikram Yoga, you will experience happiness like you've never known. That's a 110-percent guarantee.

Okay. You've been warned, and you've been invited to discover a better life, to claim your birthright as a fully realized human being. Now, can I start?

Fasten Your Seat Belts: Bikram Yoga and the Ride of Your Life

IF YOU'VE READ ANY OF THE MANY ARTICLES ABOUT ME, OR seen a TV segment such as the one on *60 Minutes*, you already know that yoga and cars are my two biggest passions. Every piece on me mentions that I own a garageful of Bentleys and Rolls-Royces. Some of what the media reports is distorted or untrue, but the part about the cars is correct: For as long as I can remember, I've been fascinated by them—the way they look, and especially the way they work. When I was a young boy in Calcutta I would stand on the street in front of my house and watch the traffic. As I spotted different cars I would call out to my mother, who was keeping an eye on me from inside, "Look! There's a Hudson! A Plymouth!"

My passion for yoga goes back just as far. Cars and yoga were my two boyhood loves, and they stayed with me as I grew up. While running my first yoga schools I simultaneously ran garages and did repairs; I even told my students which cars to buy and which ones not to buy. As I learned the workings of the human body in yoga, I taught myself the workings of the automotive body. Both run along similar principles and are easy to fix if you know how.

So it's true what they say about me: I have a garage stuffed with gleaming luxury cars, and they're beautiful. But what no one seems to realize is that they are all vintage cars that I bought as near-hopeless wrecks and restored with my own two hands. And through my teaching, and my Bikram Yoga Colleges of India that I've established here in the United States and all over the world, I do the same thing with the human vehicle. I fix the human chassis, I tune up human engines, I recharge human batteries, and I adjust human transmissions.

Practicing Hatha Yoga—and by that I mean doing my Bikram Sequence of 26 postures and two breathing exercises—is like getting a complete overhaul for your body. Full service! It cleans the gaps between your spark plugs, lubricates your joints, adjusts your fluid levels, changes the oil in your gearbox, rotates your tires and fills them to the correct psi.

The only thing that gives me as much pleasure as seeing a junked car come back to life is seeing a junked human being come back to life through yoga. I show people how to lead Rolls-Royce- and Bentley-quality lives, even those who start out on the scrap heap. I'm not a medical doctor; I'm a mechanic—the very best. You must understand that when I say I'm not a doctor, I'm not apologizing one bit. I'm *proud* not to be one of those pill-pushers in their white coats—their prescriptions don't create lasting health. I dispense yoga, the natural medicine for the human body that will heal and protect you for the rest of your life. I always say, "What's right is what works." And yoga has been proven to work for some 5,000 years.

The Purpose of This Book—and of Yoga

Like yoga itself, this book and my teachings are for everyone: the stressed-out successful career woman and mother in New York City and the overweight office worker sitting in his La-Z-Boy watching football with a 6-pack in Kansas City. But my guess is that there are two types of readers who will pick up this book. For those of you who have heard of Bikram Yoga but have never taken a class, this book is a wonderful way to introduce yourself to the practice. When you're more experienced and you've gotten instruction at one of my studios, using the book will also be a great way to maintain or supplement your practice at home; for example, on those days when you're pressed for time.

If you're already a Bikram Yoga student, my teachings here will refine your technique and deepen your understanding of what we do: how the postures and breathing exercises work, and work together, to create strength, flexibility and balance, and what's going on biologically and biomechanically in your body when you do each one of these mini tune-ups. Since I have much more room and time here than I do in class, I can explain the logic and science of the Sequence more completely, and even give you hints on practicing each posture—Bikram's Keys, I'm calling them—that go beyond the usual studio instruction.

Please understand, though, that regardless of your experience level, there's no substitute for going to a Bikram studio and working with one of our certified teachers; to make the most progress and get the greatest benefit, you absolutely need to visit Bikram's Torture Chamber.

Wait a minute. Did I just say "torture chamber"? That's right, my friend. If you don't know this already, all of my Bikram Yoga studios are heated to 105 degrees. (Later on I'll tell you how to heat your home studio to approximate these conditions.) Why do I subject you to this torture? So that you can be happy. You see, in that extreme heat we forge bodies and minds of steel. By pushing you to your limits and then beyond, I get you to understand that *there are no limits*. Everything is possible if you work hard enough and know what you're doing. Sure it's hard, but which would you rather do: suffer for 90 minutes in a Bikram class, or suffer for 90 years as you live your life without a truly healthy body and without realizing your potential?

When you practice my 26 postures, you are good for the day. You are energized, you are relaxed, you are calm. Nothing can come from outside and bother your body or your mind, I guarantee you. Such is the confidence I have in this Sequence.

But that is just the beginning. This book, like yoga, goes far beyond the execution of *asanas* (postures) and *pranayama* (breathing exercises), and even beyond my Sequence. Americans have been quick to embrace my yoga as a great way to limber up and maybe lose a big belly and tighten up a saggy butt. However, in yoga we don't deal just with the body, but also with the mind and the Spirit. You see, the goal of yoga, and life's ultimate destination, is not simply to practice—that's a means to an end. Practicing the right way is the key that starts the car and keeps it running, the essential activity that allows you to get where you want to go as a human being. And where do you need to go?

The ultimate destination of human life is Self-Realization. To define that I need to make a distinction here. When I say "Self" with a capital S, I mean the real you, the perfect you, the ultimate human potential that you carry inside you, which, I believe, is also the Divine. You have godliness in you, and so do I. That's our birthright. Our mission here on Earth is to fully inhabit or to realize the awesome potential of our true Selves. The "self" we think we are, the one spelled with a lowercase s, is just a creation of our minds, the ego. We have to break down and fight through that ego self to get to the right Self. And the only way to become a Self-Realized human being is to study and practice yoga.

We begin with the body, the physical plane. You must keep your body healthy, your temple pure—if you're sick or you die, how are you going to fulfill your destiny and experience the joy and well-being you deserve? Your body knows how to heal itself, and when you practice your Bikram Yoga, you will experience optimum, radiant health for the first time. If you're sick or run-down, or if you have some lingering, chronic condition, you'll become well, sometimes with amazing, near-miraculous speed. Maybe you're just experiencing what you think are the inevitable aches and pains of growing older, in which case you'll suddenly feel 20 years younger. And in many ways, you will be. (Aching backs and knees are my specialties; I fix them like a master mechanic fixes the suspension system or brakes on your car.) If you're already pretty healthy, in good shape, you won't believe how much *more* energy you'll have, how your physical capabilities can still expand exponentially—you'll become a superman or superwoman!

How is this possible? Yoga *asanas* rejuvenate the spine, the center of all energy in the body. If you have a good spine, you'll have a good life. The postures also strengthen the immune system; this is one of the most important ways yoga heals injuries and disease. (Prescription drugs paralyze the immune system, and they can have terrible side effects.) Through *pranayama*, the breathing exercises, we also create an essential and happy marriage between the heart and the lungs. (Most of us are in an anatomical divorce court, with the spouses bickering and spitefully refusing to cooperate.) And unlike all other types of exercise, yoga actually gives you more energy, creating a surplus rather than depleting energy or running down your batteries.

By the way, the supreme state of healthfulness you are about to enjoy has nothing to do with dieting, eating low-fat, low-carb, or raw foods, or following a vegan diet; none of that nonsense is relevant here. All you need is the yoga. You will love the beautiful slimming effects yoga has on your body; it's the natural, effective system for controlling your weight and your appetite. All this sounds pretty good, right? Of course it is! If yoga were a pill, believe me, everyone would take it. And unlike most pills, yoga has no harmful side effects—what other exercise system or medical treatment can truthfully say that?

As a human mechanic I also repair and relax your frazzled mind, making it possible for it and your body to finally work in tune with each other. Stress is one of the biggest problems we have in the United States today; not only does it ruin our quality of life, but it's also the underlying cause of many serious health conditions. Again, yoga is the natural proven remedy, for both the mental and physical reactions to stress. In addition to instructing you on the postures and breathing exercises in my

Sequence, I will also offer you some specific mental exercises to do outside the studio that will build the five qualities of mind you need to be relaxed, happy and better able to pursue your life's goals.

One of the most important of those mental qualities is concentration. Through training the body with rigor and determination we also train the mind to concentrate. The discipline of practice helps turn the mind, which for many of you is your worst enemy, into your best friend. With your new mental strength, no one and nothing outside of you will ever be able to bother you, harm you, or disrupt your mental peace. As I tell my students in class all the time: "Let no one steal your peace."

Once the body and mind are trained and joined in harmony—I call this a marriage—they can live together in harmony and be invited into the house of the Spirit. Then body, mind and Spirit form a perfect union and a complete human being. A happy, fulfilled human being. Listen to me now: If you follow my instruction and do my yoga posture Sequence to the best of your ability, you will live a better, healthier and more peaceful life. A life that's *in balance*, and most likely a longer life as well. Your attitude—your entire outlook—will improve radically along with your body and mind; your relationship to all humanity will change. That's what happens when you begin to tap your awesome potential.

Scientific studies show that most people use only 4 to 6 percent of their brains throughout their lives. Most of the brain's capability lies dormant. And in over 50 years of studying and teaching yoga, I've concluded that this is true for our bodies as well. The great Paramahansa Yogananda, author of the classic *Autobiography of a Yogi*, which is one of the most important (and best-selling) books of all time, expressed it this way:

When we begin to understand the total being that is man, we realize that he is no simple physical organism. Within him are many powers whose potential he employs in greater or lesser degree in accommodating himself to the conditions of this world. Their potential is vastly greater than the average person thinks.

However, having something doesn't mean anything if you don't know how to use it, and that includes your human potential. We all have a beautiful Rolls-Royce sitting in our garage, but some of us are forced to walk through life in the rain and snow because we simply don't know how to drive. This book will show you what the master key—Hatha Yoga—looks like, where you can find it and how to use it. It's a kind of owner's manual for your true, best Self, so you can more gracefully navigate your beautiful vehicle through the dirt roads and smooth superhighways of life. I've seen, maybe hundreds of thousands of times, how yoga practitioners realize *much more* of their hidden potential and their true power. You can actually learn to use your mind and body to 100 percent of their capacity. Then, and only then, can you access your hidden Spiritual potential, the unlimited capacity for happiness, joy and fulfillment that you have inside. Right now, you have no idea. But you will.

My Way Is the Right Way

Another thing you may have heard about me is that I criticize other yoga schools and teachers, sometimes in rough language. If I do, it is only because I care so deeply and passionately about yoga and about you, the student. I want so badly for you to receive all of yoga's fantastic, life-changing benefits—giving them to you is *my life's work*, the reason I came to this country in the first place. In this book, I'll explain why Bikram Yoga is the only true yoga being taught here in the United States, my beloved adopted home. After the "yoga boom" of the last 10 to 15 years, there are now more ridiculous, made-up flavors of so-called yoga offered here than there are flavors at Baskin-Robbins! But when practiced correctly, the yoga I teach, based on my training in India and over 50 years of practice, is the one that nourishes, the one that heals.

I'll tell you exactly how my yoga method is derived, so you can see the 5,000 years of wisdom and the real-life experience behind it. Then I'll take you through my beginning class, explaining how each component works synergistically with the others, every exercise and posture building on the previous ones and setting up the ones that follow. And I'll explain the medical benefits of each exercise, as well as the complete practice. You'll learn, as my guru, the great Bishnu Ghosh, taught me, how the regular practice of Hatha Yoga systematically diagnoses and repairs every part and every function of your body, stimulating and healing you from fingertips to toes, bones to skin, down to every single cell. As he put it: *"Yoga reenergizes, reorganizes and revitalizes."*

The Yoga of Life

After we go through our physical yoga practice together, we'll learn about yoga as a way of life and how you can practice—and benefit from—the wisdom of yoga outside the studio. In the yoga tradition we see life as divided into four separate stages, from your childhood to your last breath, and I'll explain what you need to accomplish at each stage to reach your ultimate destination. We'll also discuss how to apply this ancient life plan, modifying it when necessary, to your modern American life. For example, the third stage of life, which we call *Banaprasthya*, calls for service to others in what Americans think of as the retirement years. How might you serve the community while serving yourself as well? I've got some ideas for you, and they don't involve playing shuffleboard at some home for "seniors."

A big part of using this life plan is understanding the yoga of love and marriage, and I'll teach you about that, too. You may know that in India we often have arranged marriages—I barely knew my lovely wife, Rajashree, when my guru's son Bisu and my parents chose her for me 22 years ago! Yet our union continues to flourish after all this time. Yoga taught both of us that rather than demanding perfection from the other person and trying to change them, we needed to perfect ourselves first. That holds true no matter where you live. Only when two people make that kind of commitment can they experience the union of two souls that is marriage at its best. When they do, and when they both practice yoga, their sex life also changes for the better. Now, instead of just a body-to-body connection, they are communicating and connecting with their bodies, their minds and their souls.

The Lesson Plan

To bring you all these yoga teachings, I've organized this book into three main parts:

1. *My Story and the Meaning of Yoga:* I'm just the messenger, but it's vital that you believe and understand what I'm

telling you. So I'll start the book off by answering the question you may currently be asking yourself: *Who is Bikram, anyway, and why should I listen to him?* After I tell you about my background, including some of my life story and teaching experiences, you can decide for yourself whether I know what I'm talking about.

Then I'll explain what yoga truly is and isn't, the history and evolution of the practice—and where I fit into the yoga teaching lineage. Then I'll tell you why I believe Americans and Western civilization need yoga so much, and why the time for you to embrace it is now.

2. *The Bikram Yoga Practice.* This section discusses the evolution and dynamics of the Sequence, and includes a full explanation of and instructions for my 26 postures and two breathing exercises. In this part I will also discuss the proven medical benefits of yoga for many common ailments and health problems, including stress, obesity, insomnia, diabetes, arthritis—even cancer. Additionally, I will explain how most of what we call exercise in this country, from running to aerobics to playing sports, actually does the body more harm than good.

3. *Living Yoga.* In the last third of the book I will lay out the role the mind plays in yoga and in life, with instructions for building mental strength to go with your new and improved body. I'll tell you the role faith plays in the life of a yogi, and then detail the life plan the ancients left for us—the Four Stages of life—and how to fulfill them. I'll also talk about one of the most amazing changes that those who practice yoga experience. This comes when, having finally learned to love yourself and to see all the

good you contain, you transfer this positive outlook to the world outside your body—to everyone and everything. Now you see and feel only the boundless good and joy in life. Truly happy, you are on your way to your ultimate destination, Self-Realization.

Your Work Cut Out for You

You know what? None of this is easy. Not the physical practice, not taming the mind, not reuniting body and mind with the Spirit. In yoga, as in so many aspects of life, the right way is the hard way. I've already warned you that I'm not going to baby you—in fact, I'm going to push you farther and harder than you've ever been pushed before. At times I'm going to sound very critical of you, of American culture and the Western way of life, and believe me, I don't sugarcoat. I don't lie to make you happy. I was raised in India to believe that pointing out people's faults is to teach them, helping them to do better and be happier in the long run.

On some level, you know that criticism and bad news can actually serve you. Even though you may have been raised by parents who told you, "You're perfect just the way you are" or, "Don't worry about a thing; it's all going to work out fine." What garbage! I know you understand why I sometimes focus on problems, because you even have an expression for this: tough love. And because I care about you, I am going to be the toughest teacher you ever had.

Despite the heat, the difficulty of attaining the postures, and how hard it is to concentrate and remember all the instructions while practicing yoga, you must try with all your might to do what I am telling you the right way. Doing anything 99 percent right really means doing it 100 percent wrong! If you listen to me and follow my directions exactly, you'll get it 110 percent right. And I don't want to hear any whining, like "I'm doing the best I can." You have no idea what your best truly is—yet.

You can do it. I know it. How? Because I've seen so many bodies and lives transformed over the years that I am completely confident. It doesn't matter how old you are, what kind of shape you're in, whether you've ever done yoga before, or even if you have some kind of physical or medical challenge to deal with. With yoga, you can make wonderful change happen.

You haven't been exercising, you haven't been happy, you've made mistakes in your life up until now? Doesn't matter. The past is past; I'm offering you a new beginning. Just by taking one yoga class, you'll begin to improve your life immeasurably and change it forever. In the words of my guru, Bishnu Ghosh, who taught me from when I was just a little boy: *"It's never too late, it's never too bad, and you're never too old or too sick to start from scratch once again."*

Notice that I say "you" can do these things, and that these are "your" journeys. That's right. Your life is your responsibility, not mine. I consider each and every one of you who chooses to read this book to be one of the most intelligent people on Earth. Your decision to learn more about life through the study of yoga proves that you are prepared to act on the promise of positive change. But can I do it for you? Do I even want to do it for you? No, and no! You must accomplish this for yourself; I am just your guide, telling you how you can better achieve your goals, as my guru told me how I could achieve mine.

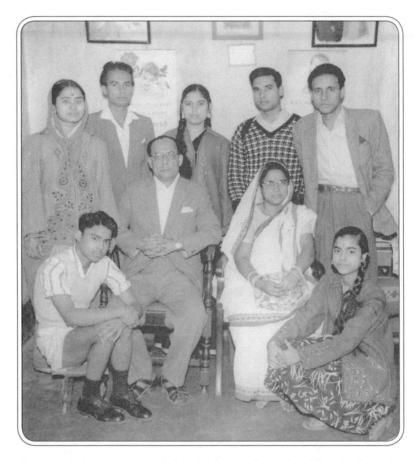

Family Photo in 1960: Top row (left to right): Maya (George's wife), my brother Asis, my sister Jayanti, me, my brother Ashim (George) Bottom Row (left to right): Bhudda, my father Kali Kinkar, my mother, Namita, my sister, Lucy

Practicing yoga is worth the effort, believe me. Even I, with all my experience, do not have the words to adequately describe the wonderful feelings, the state of living in joy, that can be yours. I consider it my duty, my mission—the reason I am here on this earth—to offer you in 21st-century America the ancient knowledge from India.

I believe that for all the triumphs of both the Eastern and Western worlds, the greatest civilization has yet to be born. This civilization will provide for all human needs: health, happiness, friendship, mental peace and a true satisfaction of living. It will be a global society connecting the genius of the West to the inner peace of the East, one in which all citizens live fully and deeply. By creating a bridge between the East and the West, I can help to bring that about and accomplish my life's goal. I already enjoy the rich material life of America, and I'm deeply grateful for my solid Indian heritage and spiritual beliefs. It's a good life; I'm a very lucky man.

By choosing to cross that bridge with me and embracing the best of both worlds, you can have it all: inner happiness and outer affluence, peace and joy, the love of yourself and others, and a love of life that you have never known.

What are you waiting for? If you want to live a healthy and fulfilling life for as long as you can, you had better get started. If you want to make this world a better place for us and our children, well, you can start by improving yourself. Only after you've worked on yourself sufficiently can you affect others, especially by sharing your knowledge and the wisdom of yoga with your family, your friends and your community.

There's a time for talk and a time for action. The time for action, for learning how to practice Bikram Yoga and understanding how yoga can transform your life is now. The way to learn is to *do*. The only way to really learn how to drive is to get behind the wheel, turn the key in the ignition, release the brake, grip the wheel tightly and put the pedal to the metal, my friend. So let's get it in gear and hit the road. Let's go!

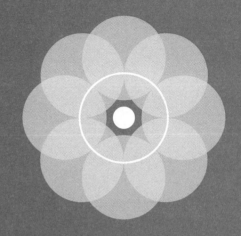

PART ONE

My Story
and
The Meaning of Yoga

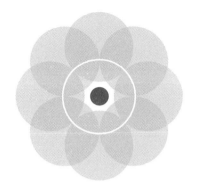

CHAPTER ONE

My Yoga Story Begins

I WAS BORN IN CALCUTTA, IN THE INDIAN STATE OF BENGAL. My father was an accountant and we were comfortable, but when I was a very little boy, there was a smallpox epidemic in Calcutta, and thousands of people died. My oldest sister, Basanti, who was 11, died within 24 hours of contracting the disease. My younger brother, Bacchu, the baby, died one day later. I suffered with the pox for eight months, and my other sister, Jayanti, suffered for more than a year, but we survived, along with Ashim, the oldest, and my second older brother, Asis. After two of her six children died, my beloved mother lost her mind to grief for a while; she just sat around, doing nothing, saying nothing. Thinking she might be happier elsewhere, my father packed everything up, and we left Calcutta to move into a big house that my family owned in the next state, Bihar, in a town called Deoghar. (My parents later had two more children: my brother Buddha, who teaches yoga in Japan, and my sister Lucy, who lives in Calcutta, India.)

Deoghar is a beautiful place, and as fate would have it, it's also considered one of the holiest places on Earth. Many of the great yogis have reached enlightenment there. Biharis speak the Hindi language, and my mother became a member of a women's club where an old master, or guru, used to teach Hindi to Bengali children like us. Because I was a noisy and energetic little boy and used to disturb my mom all the time, she had Ashim and Jayanti take me with them to the club so that I'd be out of her hair and she could cook in peace. While the others were getting their lessons, which lasted for about three hours, I would sit on the old guru's lap. Afterward the guru would say, "Your friends, your brother and your sister all study Hindi and do the chanting, so they all get candy." We had a sugar candy then that we called *prashat*. "You didn't do anything, so you are not going to get *prashat*."

I said, "Are you kidding? For three hours, I sat on your lap quietly—that's the hardest thing I ever did in my life. So I deserve candy." Even then, I had a big mouth.

The guru said, "Well, rules are rules. You've got to do something in order to earn a reward."

"What do you want me to do?" I asked him.

He just smiled, grabbed my feet and hung me upside-down with my head touching the floor, which is called *Sirsasana*, or Headstand. He also used to hold my hands and feet, and lift me up in Bow posture; at the time, I didn't realize that he was teaching me yoga *asanas*. So, every day, seven days a week, he used to hang me upside-down and make me practice various postures. It all seemed very strange to me—and, it turned out, I *still* had to learn the chanting. But I didn't really mind: I did it all for the candy.

Right after I turned six we moved back to Calcutta, to a house next door to a playground and gymnasium where all the neighborhood children played. In a club upstairs from the gym, I saw all these bodybuilders exercising. I was interested; you know how boys are naturally fascinated by muscular men. One day I went there with my friends, walked upstairs and saw them all practicing the same things that the old guru had taught me in Bihar! I bragged to one of my friends, "Hey, I can do much better than that—they're not even doing a good job." I was never a bashful person, even as a kid.

"Oh yeah?" said my friend. "Show me." So I took off my shirt, and started doing the exercises with the friend. There was a man sitting on a bed at the front of the room, and he said, "Hey, come here. What's your name?"

"Bikram," I replied. As I got closer I could see that he was a very short man; I also noticed that he had the most penetrating dark eyes I'd ever seen. They were black, and his gaze immediately struck you when it fell upon you.

"Where did you learn those things?" he asked.

"From *Punditji*," I told him. (*Punditji* means Master.) "In Deoghar."

"Show me more," he commanded.

So I showed him all the postures I knew. "A little boy doing all eighty-four postures?" he said, very surprised. "Come every day; I will teach you more."

This man was Bishnu Charan Ghosh, the youngest brother of Paramahansa Yogananda. Widely considered the greatest physical culturist to emerge in the last 500 years, he became my guru and the greatest influence in my life. I remained at his side, studied with him, and learned everything I know about yoga from him for the next 20 years. If you ask me today what it is that I do, I will tell you, "I practice my guru's wisdom."

Bishnu Ghosh was a doctor and an engineer, a professor, an athlete, a poet, a philosopher *and* a lawyer. He was internationally known; he even had lunch with President Roosevelt in the White House. Yet he also picked out poor kids begging for money on the streets and helped them realize their potential as human beings. With those piercing eyes he had a special kind of sight that instantly revealed to him what any person was meant to do in this world, where their true talents lay, and how their Karma Yoga could be fulfilled. And I was blessed that he saw something special in me.

My guru loved me unconditionally, but his love for me was not coddling, not the kind that offers excuses. Instead, it was challenging. There was no room for weakness. No room for smoking, drinking or fooling around. He beat me like a hammer all my life, so that nobody could ever make a scratch on my body, on my mind or on my soul. He made me bulletproof, cold-proof, fireproof, windproof, emotion-proof, sex-proof, money-proof, stress-proof—everything-proof! This was not an easy job for either of us, you understand, but that's where the discipline of yoga comes in.

How tough was he? My guru used to hang a very large, very sharp sword on the wall of his school, and threaten to cut off our heads when he saw that we weren't trying hard enough. I never heard of him following through on this threat, but I chose not to question the sincerity of his words. Did I ever believe for one second of my life that my beloved guru would do anything to harm me directly? No. Did his tactics work? Oh, yes.

My guru motivated us by screaming his way through our lives. Nothing we did, no matter how perfect, was ever good enough. He would refuse to eat until I had performed a posture to his satisfaction, constantly sending back the reheated plate of food his wife would send him until I finally—in the wee hours of the morning, with my legs shaking and foam dripping out of my mouth—did a particular *asana* to his standards. When you are at the very brink of physical, mental and emotional exhaustion, and some raving madman swinging a razor-sharp sword is screaming at you so loudly that your hair is blown back by the force of his voice, believe me, you listen. Now, every time I want to quit, compromise or just get up and leave, my guru is there with his sword, acting like the angriest yogi on Earth. I miss him so much; you have no idea.

Not only did I have one of the world's greatest gurus, I was also fortunate to have been educated at one of the great *ashrams*, or schools—the Ram Krishna Mission, also in Deoghar. Ram Krishna was the guru of Swami Vivekenanda, the first Indian yogi to bring the message of Self-Realization to the United States, in 1893. The training I received at the Mission was a million times harder than the intensive yoga teacher training I currently dish out. Let me give you an idea of a typical day.

Dong, dong, dong, dong, the bell rings at 4:30 in the morning. The other boys and I get up, splash a little water on our faces, and go outside to start gardening. Little kids gardening! At 4:30 in the morning no less! Then we go to the shed and clean up the cow dung to help the man who milked the cows. After that, we wash up and get to play either cricket or football (which Americans call soccer). Then we shower.

At exactly 6:45 we go to the temple to chant and pray in Sanskrit. (I was never any good at this because I still only spoke Bengali, which is completely different.) After the temple chanting, it's time for breakfast. In America, this would be a full day already, but we haven't even had our first meal. After breakfast, we study all the usual academic subjects from 8 until 11:30 a.m., when we break for lunch.

After lunch, we study until 3:30 p.m. Then we can go play or do some more gardening for a half an hour. Next we go to the temple again for another 45 minutes of chanting and meditation, then we study in our rooms until dinnertime. After dinner, it's back to the dorm and in bed by 8:30. Soon it's 4:30, and we hear that *dong, dong, dong,* and we start all over again. There was no escape, not even any variation: Our whole lives were spent entirely within the boundaries of the school property.

During my time at the *ashram* I continued to study Hatha Yoga and weight lifting with Bishnu Ghosh, competing successfully in both areas. At the age of 13 I became the youngest person ever to win the All-India Yoga Asana Championship, and I went on to win it the next two years as well.

I also started breaking records as a weight lifter. I loved weight lifting; I wanted to be a world-famous athlete, like Pelé, the great soccer player. Then, one day when I was 18, I was practicing and a spotter dropped a 380-pound weight on my knee, pulverizing it. (I often tell my students, "You can mess with the gods, but don't mess with the knees.")

Effectively a cripple, I was told by doctors I would never walk again. Some of them wanted to amputate my leg below the knee, and others said they would try to rebuild my knee with stainless steel. For months my sister had to carry me to the bathroom. I couldn't take the idea of being lame for the rest of my life, and I actually thought about killing myself. Instead, I called my guru. I limped back to him, and he saved me. He had two huge bodybuilders force my legs—including the shattered knee—into Lotus position. If you are familiar with this cross-legged position you know it requires great flexibility of the knees. The pain was unbelievable. I'd bite my finger or a stick, and I'd pass out. But after six months I could do it myself. It was nothing less than a miracle, and this inspired me to become a yoga teacher.

When I or any other sick or injured person came to see him, my guru would prescribe what the patient should do 24 hours a day, according to that person's condition. He'd make a chart, telling the person what to eat and what not to eat, and he would prescribe specific yoga postures as well. If the patient had a back problem, postures focusing on the spine would be prescribed. Postures focusing on the kidneys would be prescribed for diabetics, and so on. Hundreds of people would wait in line to see him. Remember, this was in India, a very poor country where people cannot afford to go to the hospital. Yoga was used as a means of curing the sick, as well as preventing illness. After figuring out which postures he wanted a patient to do, my guru would call in me or one of his other disciples. Our job was to take the patient into another room and teach him or her how to do the postures correctly. So each patient received the individual attention of a yoga teacher.

However, that tradition began to change in March 1965, when my guru sent me to Bombay. There I taught yoga to the family of

Mr. S. P. Jain, a disciple of my guru and a very wealthy man who owned many magazines and newspapers, including the *Times of India*. He had five sons and many of them had health problems, including one who suffered from epilepsy. I lived with them and tried to heal them for over a year. At the same time, I was treating patients at several hospitals as well as a polio clinic. It wasn't easy, believe me, but my guru had given me no choice.

People who know me understand that the two dominant aspects of my personality are best represented by the English bulldog and the Bengal tiger. With English bulldog determination and Bengal tiger strength, I will always do my best to perform my Karma Yoga, or life's work—the duty that my guru charged me with—to teach yoga to as many people as possible.

But in Bombay I found there were more sick people in need of my help than I could possibly treat; at times there would be 100 people waiting to see me, men, women and children—even some 80-year-olds. They had all kinds of medical problems, mostly common ones: spinal problems, arthritis, heart problems, diabetes, thyroid problems, neurological diseases. But if I treated them one-on-one, I could see only 15 people a day! I thought that if there was some way I could teach everyone the right postures in the correct order, no matter what their disease or condition, then I could teach in groups and help more people. If penicillin worked on so many kinds of infections, couldn't one yoga prescription be used that way, too? What's more, yoga would work as preventive medicine as well.

This was a totally different approach from the single teacher–single student method that had been the norm for thousands of years. At first my guru opposed this idea. He told me it was impossible to help everyone with just one prescription. Nevertheless, I

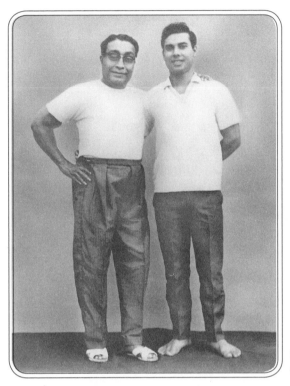

My guru, Bishnu Charan
Ghosh and me, 1965

began developing my Sequence of 26 postures, and in time, as he
saw the beneficial effects of the postures on all who came to my
class, he was won over and ended up being the strongest sup-
porter of my revolutionary Sequence. (Here I would also like to
thank and honor my guru's son, Biswanath (Bisu) Ghosh. He inspired me when I first went to work in Bombay and he made many
sacrifices in his life so that I could become who I am today.)

Around this time I met Shirley MacLaine, a Hollywood ac-
tress and spiritual seeker. We were at a party given by the movie
actor Dev Anand (the Gregory Peck of India) in Juhu Beach. We
sat together on the beach and talked for an hour. I was a movie
buff and had seen nearly all of her films. She shared with me how

she had actually left Hollywood to live in India in search of the truth of life. I told her, "You are in the wrong place. You won't find the truth in India. Go back to Hollywood, sing, dance and entertain the people; that's your duty, your Karma Yoga. When the time is right, India will come to you."

She responded by saying, "Promise me you'll come to America." She said that her country needed someone like me and needed yoga. Soon my guru would make it clear to me that she was right: Just as it is Shirley's job to entertain, it's my job to help as many people as possible by sharing my Indian heritage and the wisdom passed down over the centuries.

In February 1970 I left India and went to Japan, for what was supposed to be six months, to take care of some things there for my guru. I didn't want to go—I was a king in Bombay! But when your guru tells you to do something, you have to do it. That's it. You have no choice. As I was about to get on the plane at Calcutta Airport, my guru took my hand and told me something, in English, which he never spoke. "Promise me you will complete my incomplete job," he said. He meant bringing yoga to the rest of the world, to the West and America. And I replied, "Yes, I promise. I will." Forty years later I'm here in the United States, still performing my Karma Yoga by fixing broken bodies and screw-loose brains.

When Bishnu Ghosh bound me in that oath, I had no way of knowing it would be the last time we spoke. Soon thereafter my guru talked to all his family and friends, gave them his blessings, and said that he would soon take his rest. He then performed *mahasamadhi*, withdrawing his Spirit from his body and leaving this Earth at the age of 67.

Looking back, I can't help feeling sad, mostly because I miss him every second of every day with every ounce of my heart. But

I'm also sad because I forgot to ask him how long I am supposed to continue teaching Hatha Yoga to fulfill my Karma Yoga! Do I have to keep doing this for my entire life? With no guru to answer me, I have to conclude that the answer is yes. To which I say, "No problem!"

In Tokyo, I taught seven days a week; I went out only on Sunday nights, to see a movie and eat out. Only once a week did I see the sky and the stars. I quickly became a superstar, teaching the Imperial family and all the famous actors and actresses. Seven months after I got there, I opened my *second* school, in the richest, trendiest part of the city—like the area around Rodeo Drive in Beverly Hills. During my time there, I healed the Japanese politician Mr. Kakuei Tanaka (who would later become prime minister), of cerebral thrombosis. I was also able to participate in studies at Tokyo University Hospital that helped to prove many of yoga's medical benefits. After a couple of years I began teaching in Hawaii as well, splitting my time between Tokyo and Honolulu. It was in Hawaii that my life took another fantastic turn.

On one of my trips there I was summoned to Oahu, where I was met by the governor of Hawaii and a bevy of Secret Service agents. I was whisked away in a stretch limousine to a hotel, where, on the sixth floor, I was presented to U.S. president Richard Nixon. He was suffering from advanced thrombophlebitis in his left leg, lying in bed in excruciating pain and unable to walk. It seems Mr. Tanaka had recommended me to him or to his people. I said, "Piece of cake. Bring me some Epsom salts."

I filled the bathtub and I gave President Nixon a hydropathic treatment; this is part of the yoga therapy that I was taught, which I give my private patients. It's yoga, but in a bathtub. I gave him six treatments in three days, and by the next morning he was comfortable and able to walk to the bathroom, brush his teeth, and shave. There was no pain; it was gone and would never return.

Several days later we met at the airport to say good-bye. President Nixon had to return to Washington, D.C., on Air Force One, and I was returning to Tokyo. He was very grateful and invited me back to D.C. with him. "No, thank you," I replied. "I must return to my work in Tokyo." The president handed me an envelope, which I put in my pocket and promptly forgot about. I handed him a 20-minute cassette with yoga instructions. "Do this every day," I told him, "and you will never even remember which leg was the bad one."

When I got back to Tokyo, the U.S. ambassador met me at the airport. "Did the president give you anything before you left?" he asked. I remembered the envelope, which was still unopened in my pocket. I showed it to him. "Open it," he said.

It was my green card, my ticket to live permanently in America, for which I had never even applied!

In July 1973 I came to Los Angeles, where I've lived and taught ever since. With some help from friends, I was soon able to open my own school. For months I slept at the school, even though I had an apartment: I'd fall asleep on the floor with a towel on top of me at 4:30 in the morning. By 7:00 I was up, shaved and showered before starting to teach class. That is what life is. The hard way, not the easy way.

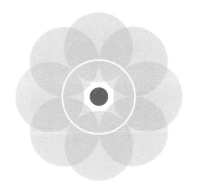

CHAPTER TWO

What Is Yoga? Defining the Practice

All creation is governed by law. The ones which manifest in the outer universe, discoverable by scientists, are called natural laws. But there are subtler laws ruling the realms of consciousness which can be known only through the inner science of yoga.

—Sri Yukteswar

YOU KNOW, FOR THE FIRST TWO YEARS THAT I TAUGHT IN THE United States, before I opened my school in Beverly Hills in July of 1973, I never charged anyone a dime to take my classes. I thought that all yoga schools had to be free because in India they're like temples. I never paid my guru one penny. (I did sweep the floors and do other things to help him.) After about eight months, Shirley MacLaine, with whom I had reconnected, explained to me that I needed to charge for sharing this wisdom. "Bikram," she said, "this is not India. This is not Calcutta. This is Beverly Hills; you're in America now. When in Rome you must do as the Romans do."

"But if I ask for money," I protested, "then I'm a false yogi, a fraud."

"In America, if you don't charge money," Shirley told me, "people won't respect you. They'll think you're full of it." I was so new to this country, I didn't even know what she meant by "full of it." Full of what? I know now, though, believe me. Anyway, she hired a manager for me and a secretary, Jackie. If you wanted to take my class, you had to pay Jackie three dollars. So Shirley started it. Don't blame me. I arrived in America as a holy, spiritual, innocent, virginal yogi. Why are you laughing? It's true!

Okay, I knew nothing about how things were done in America. But Americans knew even less about yoga. When I started teaching here, most people didn't know the difference between yoga and yogurt. As I say that now, though, it occurs to me that you might not know the difference either! So much bad information has been accepted in this country, and there is so much fake yoga being taught, that I really need to give you an explanation of what true yoga is and the history and the meaning of this fantastic thing. Let me give you a clear, definitive answer to the question What is yoga?

In Sanskrit, the ancient root language of the great works of Indian philosophy, the word *yuj* means "to join." The term "yoga" comes from that word, and symbolizes union—a joining, or a marriage. Who is getting married here? You are, my friend. Through the physical practice of yoga, you integrate your body and mind in a perfect union. Then, in another marriage, or union, you can merge your body and mind with the godliness, or Spirit, that naturally exists in you and become a whole, fully realized human being.

Yoga is the science of living life correctly so we can get to that point, our ultimate destination. The great yogis of India have been perfecting that science for roughly 5,000 years. Why do I call it a science? Science helps us understand the physical world; that's what physics, chemistry and mathematics attempt to do. Yoga helps us understand not just the physical body but also the mind and the Spirit. Yoga helps us understand nature; nature helps us understand the voice of our spirit, or God. Yoga is universal and 100 percent natural—it's the science of life.

Patanjali is perhaps the greatest of those ancient sages, the "father of yoga." About 4,700 years ago he researched the work of all the previous yogis and he devised the original 84 *asanas*. He and the other great ancients originally created the postures as a way of preparing the body so it could sit still in meditation. Through that practice, they saw that we can improve our powers of concentration, the quality we all need to recognize and achieve our Karma Yoga and Self-Realization.

When those first yogis were sitting there, though, attempting to meditate, their minds would start telling them that their knees were complaining, distracting them from their meditation with these physical sensations. No wonder the yogis' first achievement was 14 seated postures, and out of these, *Padmasana*, the cross-legged Lotus position, was found to be the most conducive to meditation. When you sit in Lotus Pose, blood is impeded from reaching your body below the waistline; it's like the gate or dam is closed. This serves as a natural local anesthesia, dulling the pain receptors so the aches of the lower body cease to demand the attention of the meditator's mind. Calm body, calm mind.

According to some accounts, devising these 14 postures alone may have taken thousands of years. The remainder of the classical 84 postures was developed afterward, to prepare the rest of the body and allow it to be calm and still as well. This physical aspect of yoga is called Hatha Yoga. Why is it called that? In Sanskrit, *Ha* means "Sun" and *Tha* means "Moon." In Nature, there is a strong, symbiotic relationship between the two, a balance between these two powerful astronomical forces. You can see this communion in the rising and falling of the tides in the ocean, which follow the gravitational force between Earth and the Moon.

Every two weeks we alternate between a full moon and a new moon. Out of the Sun's and the Moon's alternating forces comes energy, or *prana*. This life force animates our planet. During the time of the full moon, for example, the energy of every human being's body is drawn up by this intensified gravitational pull. If you suddenly experience pain in your knee, back or ankle, it is very likely to be within one day of the full moon. This especially affects older people who suffer from such ailments as rheumatism and bursitis because they have less energy and are less able to physically resist the pull of the Moon.

So as you can see, the union between the Sun and the Moon maintains the balance of life on Earth. This marriage also reflects and maintains the perfect balance, or symmetry, of the human body. Think about it: We have two arms, two legs, two eyes, two ears, two kidneys, two lobes in our brains. So many parts of the human body are symmetrical and dual. Why? Balance. One part, or region, belongs to the Sun, and one to the Moon—*Ha* and *Tha*. Balance means health. Yoga creates balance; that's how it heals. Disease is an imbalance, often of body chemistry—a biochemical imbalance.

What many people don't realize, though, is that this physical aspect is really only a small part of what I teach. Hatha Yoga is a fraction of yoga. *Asanas*, the postures, are a fraction of Hatha Yoga. Before I get you to leap from the frying pan of theory into the fire of my practice, you must understand that the ancient masters actually identified eight different forms of yoga. Called Karma Yoga, Hatha Yoga, Raja Yoga, Vedanta Yoga, Bhakti Yoga, Mantra Yoga, Jnana Yoga, and Laya Yoga, they are all tools for a happy life. Together, they comprise every conceivable aspect of existence. Here are explanations of the eight yoga forms.

1. *Karma Yoga:* Work and duty. This is the most important of all. The Earth is like a factory, and you are here to do your job: working to fulfill your destiny. You must do it honestly, trying the right way, and you must do it *on time*, before you die. Both your actions and the results of those actions are *karma*. Helping and serving others on this path is one important way to transcend the ego-based self spelled with the lowercase *s* and realize the higher Self spelled with the uppercase *S*.

2. *Hatha Yoga:* Physical practice, including *asanas* and *pranayama*. You scientifically create balance and health within the body, then maintain it.

3. *Raja Yoga:* Mental processes and rational thought; the intellect. You use your mind to get the right guidance, bringing your emotions under control and putting less emphasis on sensory, external perceptions. *Raja* means "royal," and this introspective, meditative form of yoga is sometimes called the royal path.

4. *Vedanta Yoga:* Philosophical grounding, including the sharing of thoughts and ideas. This form of yoga helps

you to understand your purpose and destination. One of its most essential teachings is that we humans are divine, that "the individual is none other than God." *Veda* can be translated as "knowledge," and *anta* means "end"; *Vedanta* is an applied philosophy or practice—a way of knowing through experience—that goes beyond where mere knowledge ends.

5. *Bhakti Yoga:* Devotional practice. Here the yogi seeks out and comes to see the Divine in all people and in all creations of the universe. This form of yoga includes formal worship, praying and surrender to God. Jesus and Gandhi, for example, were *bhakti* yogis who showed their loving devotion in every single action and thought of their daily lives.

6. *Mantra Yoga:* Chanting and using sound to help achieve peace and calm. A mantra is a word or phrase that you chant or repeat silently to yourself when meditating (doing this is called *japa*). *Mantra* Yoga helps you to set your intention and to focus your attention. But it is also very much like a prayer, calling forth Divine power, so it aids in devotion as well (in the beginning *mantras* were taken only from the Vedas or scriptures). The importance of *mantra* comes from the ancient belief that the universe came to be created through sound.

7. *Jnana Yoga:* The way of attained wisdom; often the path of a sage or scholar. (Literally, *Jnana* means "knowledge"; *Ajnana* means "ignorance.") This form of yoga requires not just countless years of study but also great strength of will; it is considered a very advanced path, for more experienced yogis rather than the masses.

8. *Laya Yoga:* The imagination, esoteric ideas and abstract thought. What is the fifth dimension? What if there is life on Jupiter? These are questions for which there are not yet any definitive answers. *Laya* Yoga concentrates on the mind's ultimate capabilities and, to reach them, yogis must learn to break down ordinary limitations and mental conditioning. This often involves meditation and tapping into the *chakras*, the cosmic energy centers in the human body.

While I have listed them separately, these forms of yoga are actually completely simultaneous, interdependent and circular in nature. They are eight in one. Let me explain using myself as an example.

✦ My Karma Yoga is to help bring happiness, success and peace into your life with the knowledge I was given.

✦ To perform my Karma Yoga successfully, I have to first maintain a healthy body, which is why I practice Hatha Yoga. This heals, strengthens and purifies my body for Raja Yoga, the practice of controlling the mind. (The clear thinking and decision making that led me to begin practicing in the first place is also Raja Yoga, the use of my conscious mind. Your reading this book, and the concentration required, are Raja Yoga as well.)

✦ Only by controlling the mind in Raja Yoga can I achieve the meditative state I need to focus on my Karma Yoga: bringing you the knowledge I was given. That knowledge assumes the forms of Jnana Yoga, the way of wisdom and understanding, and Laya Yoga, the way of esoteric knowledge, metaphysics and spiritual teaching.

◆   When I was young I began to join my body, mind and spirit using Bhakti Yoga, devotional yoga (though I don't practice this any longer).

◆   Bhakti Yoga can be helped along by singing, chanting or prayer, which are all forms of Mantra Yoga, the yoga of sound.

◆   Even before my guru gave me my mantra, I had to understand the relationship between Spirit, body and mind, and how to bridge the gaps between them. To do that I needed Vedanta Yoga, which deals with the philosophy of human life. He taught Vedanta Yoga to me, and now I am writing this book as a form of Vedanta Yoga to teach you—and so the circle continues.

This may sound complicated; I know it's a lot to absorb. But the essence is simple, and the first three steps form the foundation. Karma Yoga is number one; nothing is more important in your life, in my life or in this world than fulfilling your cosmic duty. This is what maintains balance and harmony in the universe. To perform your Karma Yoga, you must first practice Hatha Yoga with your body, which in turn relies upon the successful practice of Raja Yoga, using the mind. Through Raja and Hatha we get to Karma, carrying out our life's responsibilities and realizing our souls.

One of the greatest epics ever written is the *Mahabharata*, the story of Lord Krishna and Arjun, which is the original story of Karma Yoga. It's unbelievably long; it would take years for most people to finish reading it. I'll just cut to the chase, and tell you what happens: Arjun is the hero, a great warrior; his name means "shining" or "silver." An archer, he is the general of the forces for good on the eve of a great battle. The great god Lord Krishna is

Arjun's brother-in-law, chariot driver and adviser. Arjun doesn't want to fight this battle because of the slaughter he knows will follow, and because he knows that among the enemy are many of his relatives. The dialogue that ensues between the two men is called the *Bhagavad Gita,* or *The Song of God.*

Facing this great moral crisis, Arjun is told by Krishna that his true duty lies in the struggle for what is right, whatever the personal loss or reward, and that doing this duty supersedes every other possible action in human life, be it spiritual or material. Krishna tells him, "You have no choice. And if others die as a result of your right actions, it is a holy death." This story illustrates the eternal balance of the universe that must be maintained by the fulfillment of Karma Yoga.

All of this rests on understanding and, most important, believing with your whole being in the philosophy, or Vedanta, of life: knowing why you are here and that your birthright and ultimate goal is Self-Realization. When you truly believe in what you do, you are much more likely to accomplish it, because you *want* to do it. The different forms of yoga are the tools in your toolbox, the means to living a happy and fulfilled life. You always need the proper tools. Even if you really and sincerely want to build a house, even if you *totally* understand why this house is needed, without a hammer and saw it'll never get built. The tools that help you build your spiritual house, for example, are Bhakti Yoga, the way of devotion, and Mantra Yoga, the way of voice and sound.

Now that you know what yoga's really made of, as it were, and where it came from, we can move forward. You can never start your journey if you don't know your destination. Just as important, however, is to know *why* you are doing something, so later in this book—after we've explored Hatha Yoga, all its great health benefits, and my Sequence fully—I will explain more about the specific ways we achieve Self-Realization. That journey, the ride of your life, can only take place once all the parts of yoga are installed in your car's engine, and the engine is firing away on all cylinders.

Myths and Madness: Clearing Away Confusion about Yoga

First, though, let me continue to define yoga by telling you a few things that yoga is *not*.

- ◆ *Yoga is not a diet.* I swear, I don't understand the way people eat in this country. If you're not eating like pigs, then you are eating like goats, munching raw foods or organic foods because you think it will make you healthy. But because of the shape most of your digestive systems are in, you can't process that food anyway, especially raw food. If your engine is broken, what difference does it make what kind of gas you put in your tank? I'll talk more later about food and obesity; my point here is that eating some trendy California way or avoiding carbs isn't a requirement or even relevant. I love to eat at McDonald's, and my favorite food is cheesecake with blueberries on top. My students who know that bring it to me all the time. I love it—so don't worry, yoga is not about eating one "right way."

- ◆ *Yoga is not deprivation.* No one's asking you to give up all your worldly possessions and go sleep on the floor of a mud hut somewhere in the Himalayas. However you choose to live your life is perfectly all right.

You must give up some bad habits, though, to stop doing things that are wrong for you. Many of these things are simply habits of mind, or *mudra*, negative attitudes that are easy to fall into. Others are negative, harmful actions, toward others and yourself. Personally, I have never smoked anything, drunk any alcohol or had one cup of tea or coffee in my life. At my wedding, people wanted me to drink Champagne, but I didn't taste it. I remember another time a student of mine offered me something to smoke at my birthday party.

"What the hell is this?" I asked, looking at the funny little cigarette.

He looked at me incredulously. "Oh my god, Bikram, you don't smoke pot?"

I told him, "In India, the janitors, the people who sweep the streets, smoke this so they can get through their day and do their job. They call it *ganja*. Why do you want to smoke this?"

"But Bikram," he said, "you don't know what you're missing!"

"Oh no," I replied, "you don't know what *you're* missing by not living a clean, decent life."

So you have some bad habits. So what? It's no big deal. Change them. When you become a real yogi, and you start to feel what true health, energy and love of yourself and life are like, it will be easy to drop those things and walk away. Once you see the right way, it will be easy for you to leave the wrong behind. Imagine you see a cup of hot tea on a table in front of you. The cup is turned so the handle is on the far side of the cup, and you can't see it. So you grab the cup, burn your hand, and *then* you see the handle. After this experience, are you going to hold the cup the same way next time, every time? No. So why would you continue to do yourself harm by indulging in bad habits? That makes no sense.

This is not a question of morality. It's a duty, a responsibility. Your job is to keep your body clean and protect it from harm. This harm you must avoid also includes marking, tattooing or piercing the body. You see, when people do such foolish things, they are looking for change externally when they really should be looking internally. If I became president I would make tattoos illegal! It's ignorant to ruin the divine beauty of your own body that way, and you have no right to do it. Just like you have no right to put cocaine in your body. Why? Because that body doesn't belong to you; it's the holy temple of your *atma*, the soul, or Spirit. You have no right to vandalize the body in these ways.

◆ *Yoga is not a religion.* Listen, I come from one of the most religious countries that ever existed and I have never been to a temple to worship in my entire life. Why? Because I never believed in it. People look at statues, lifeless hunks of stone and plaster, and they pray to them, hoping that the statue is really listening to them—I just don't buy it. And if this is all about God, why do so many people go to church, mosque or temple and then give money? Do you really think you can bribe God? What does God need money for, anyway? Worst of all, religion has been misused throughout human history. Differences in religious beliefs, often amplified by differences in skin color, caste or ethnicity, have created walls between countries, between brothers and sisters and in our own hearts. That's the biggest thing I've got against organized religion. My duty in this life is simply this: to break down walls between people and nations, men and women, East and West.

I worship in a different temple: my body. There is something inside this temple, an animating force that makes my flesh move and speak, that moves me toward my Karma Yoga. What is this mystical but everyday magic? It is the *atma*, the soul. You can also call it the Spirit, or the true Self. This is God, and God lives in the house of our bodies. We are all Gods and Goddesses. Getting down on your knees, wearing elaborate robes or building a $40 million church doesn't bring you any closer to the Divine that lives within us all.

So when you ask me if I believe in God, I will never be able to answer with a simple yes or no. I'm going to say, "Yes, I do, because I believe in myself, and I am God. I believe in you, too, because you are my God." The only danger in this belief comes when we refuse to recognize everyone else as an expression of the Divine and see only ourselves that way. If you think you have more of God within you than anyone else, you're in real trouble, my friend. And so is the world we live in.

In the West today, and really around the planet, there's a new religion, consumerism, that is holding us back from our birthright of happiness. When people are more concerned with the car they drive or the clothes they wear than the lives of their global brothers and sisters, then something is terribly wrong. It's about money from the day you're born till the day you die. Materialism is the number one problem in the West today, because it's the opposite of Spiritualism.

Yoga provides us with positive, useful tools to help us realize the God within us and achieve real liberation and perfection of the soul. That is not religion, but rather Spirituality. Spirit is the expression of God through the medium of our human body. The body is the temple of the living Spirit and provides a home for our individual expression of God. When we don't revere and treat the physical body properly, it becomes a bad home, so to speak; in essence we are encouraging the Spirit to leave. Nobody sets out to make their bodies ill-prepared to house their Spirit. It's usually just slow, continuous and mindless abuse over the course of time. Little by little, day by day, the Spirit becomes very unhappy as the body suffers a slow death by poison. It doesn't have to be this way.

The best way to reverse this downward spiral is to first agree that the human body is the temple of the living Spirit. Second, you must be willing to accept responsibility for cleaning up your "house" and providing the level of accommodation that is fit for your soul. And third, you must be willing to replace bad habits with good ones. And you can accomplish all three of these things through Hatha Yoga, or physical yoga.

Only if you can establish real faith in your Self, and faith in all people, do you truly have the right to claim faith in God. By slowly changing all of your bad habits, by only making choices that serve to make you a better human being, you can begin to make the positive changes that will reestablish faith in your Self. You know what is right and what is wrong for you in your life; you just need to develop the moral strength necessary to see it through.

Dangerous Games

*RUNNING, JUMPING, WORKING OUT,
AEROBICIZING, BALL PLAYING AND OTHER
BODY KILLING FORMS OF "EXERCISE"*

While we're on the subject of what yoga is *not*, let me break some more news that will shock most of my readers: Yoga is not an "exercise" or a "workout," and what you think of as exercise isn't good for you.

Here's the biggest difference between exercise and yoga: The purpose of what Americans think of as exercise is to reach a sports or fitness goal, regardless of cost to the body. The purpose of yoga is to heal, using the body to create health. That's its *dharma*, its nature. Just like fire's *dharma* is to burn, and the wind's *dharma* is to blow, the function and destiny of yoga is to heal. And fitness is merely a by-product of this health-building process.

I've told you that I fix junked cars and junked bodies. Where do you think those bodies come from? The gym. The jogging trail. The aerobics studio. And sometimes, from yoga studios run by people who don't know what they're doing. I honestly don't know which is worse—the way so many Americans ruin their bodies by not using them at all, or the way they ruin their bodies by blindly running around "exercising" and playing sports. I tell my students, "No barbells, no dumbbells, no racket." Games are okay for children, for recreation and to teach them sportsmanship. But after that, you must give up trying to put a little round ball in a hole all the time.

Why do I say that? First, the repeated impact from running, playing sports, and taking aerobics classes—and even dancing—results in abnormal wear of the joints and (as I discuss in depth later) damage to the spine and nervous system. You may get a 5 percent benefit; for example, your legs will get stronger. But you are doing 95 percent harm. Second, the combined impact and repeated limited motions inherent in these kinds of activities, from weight lifting to tennis and everything in between, create overuse injuries, such as destroyed cartilage, impingements and muscle tears. Third, many of these so-called exercises call for unnatural motions; their only purpose lies in playing some ridiculous game. Do you think that's what you were put on earth to do? No.

Running, jogging, biking and the like are always touted for their aerobic benefit, but this isn't entirely true. "Aerobic exercise" means maintaining a sufficient oxygen level in the bloodstream to support the work the body is attempting to perform. So the benefit isn't an optimum oxygen level, or the highest level possible for the human body, but only the level required for that particular activity. So no matter how fast you run, how many stairs you climb, how long you spin or how far you walk, if you haven't trained your lungs with yogic breathing exercises and you don't challenge them with yoga *asanas*, you're not getting the highest possible benefit—and you may be causing harm to your body.

Let's imagine that your lungs are a glass that holds one pint of water. When you start to exercise, you begin to fill the glass. After a few minutes the glass becomes full, but you continue to exercise and the water overflows. The glass can hold only so much, and once you have filled it to capacity, you can't force any more water in there. That's the way it is when you do aerobic exercise; your lungs have only so much capacity, so you can fill them only so much. Yoga gives you a gallon jug for lungs instead of that pint glass—you follow me?

There is also some cardiovascular benefit to what passes for exercise here, but again it's limited. Running or working out will get your heart rate up and the blood pumping a little more than usual, but when that happens the blood is being distributed equally throughout your entire body, so the therapeutic effect on each part is minimal. It's nothing compared to the blood flow you create in Hatha Yoga through the extension and compression of the veins and arteries in one specific part of the body, or wringing out individual organs and then flooding them with blood, as I will describe in chapter 5.

Face it, most of what people call exercise these days would qualify as cruelty to animals. The proof can be seen in the people who pursue these things the most intensely: Look at professional athletes and dancers; after just a few years, they end up crippled with broken bodies that can't play or perform anymore. They're like yellow cabs in New York City: They've been driven too much, too hard, in too short a time. Then they have to come to Bikram's Torture Chamber and do yoga with me just so they can walk. The worst students in my class are always world-champion athletes. I once taught Wayne Collette, who was the gold medalist in the 400 meters at the Munich Olympics in 1972. A big, 6-foot, 6-inch, muscular guy with a beautiful body, he came to my class, fell down during the standing postures about 23 times, then threw up. Meanwhile next to him was a 72-year-old lady doing the postures perfectly. You see, Wayne ran too hard for too long, ruining his body, and Nature doesn't accept that.

A notch down the intensity scale are the "hard-core" amateur athletes. Very often, people who try to keep in shape by doing all these unnatural exercises end up with serious physical problems, including back injuries. All that jumping around, kicking the legs in unnatural directions and arm-flailing puts extreme pressure on the spine, wrists, elbows and shoulder joints.

Last but not least, let's take a hard look at you, my friend. Why do you think you have pulled muscles, shin splints, tennis elbow, sprained ankles, sciatica and other ailments? Your body is telling you that what you are doing for exercise is *WRONG*. And when you start to break down, where do you go for answers? To the so-called experts, including doctors, exercise physiologists and dime-store trainers at your local gym. Did you know that with absolutely no previous experience in sports or exercise, anyone with a pulse and a checkbook can get certified as a "physical trainer" in a single weekend? What does that person know? Would you go to a demolition-derby driver to fix your broken car?

"But Bikram," you say, "the exercise I'm doing makes me feel good. Isn't that a good thing?" Sure, it makes you feel good temporarily, because your body craves movement and activity. But sports and commonly accepted forms of "exercise" do not give you what you need. Real exercise means stretching, the simultaneous contraction and elongation of the muscles, which builds strength and flexibility. There's no jarring, repetitive impact, no unnatural motions. That's why my guru said: "Yoga maintains youth long. It keeps the body full of vitality, immune to diseases, even at old, old age."

Let's break it down in a more businesslike way; we'll do a cost-benefit analysis. Your time is valuable, your body is valuable, and you are valuable. Hatha Yoga will maximize your time and effort by doing the most good in the shortest amount of time. When practiced intelligently, yoga has no negative side effects, while other exercises damage you. You tell me, what is the best investment?

I know many of you enjoy playing your sports; at the very least, you must do *both*, adding yoga to whatever activities you currently do. Don't just take my word for it; listen to my friend, long-time student and one of the greatest athletes in the history of American sports, Kareem Abdul-Jabbar. When he first came to me in the early 1980s he had already been punishing his body for 13 years in the National Basketball Association. I told him that by practicing with me he would be able to keep playing for another five years—and he laughed out loud. But he came to class faithfully and he ended up playing for more than seven years, until he was 42, which is practically unheard of in the world of professional sports; that's considered advanced old age! And during his last seasons, his team, the Los Angeles Lakers, won the NBA championship three times. Here are his words:

> *I first learned about yoga while reading the book* Autobiography of a Yogi, *and that led me to my first Hatha Yoga teacher, Nawana Davis, in 1978. I went to her class for a few months on and off during the basketball off-season. Then, in 1982 I was introduced to Bikram. I started to go to his class and I have practiced yoga in some form ever since. I truly believe that it helped to prolong my career and kept me from getting serious injuries. The stretching aspect of yoga perfectly complements the strength training and cardiovascular endurance that are so well covered in traditional sports workouts. I've encouraged my parents and children, along with other athletes, to learn about yoga and incorporate it into their training regimens.*
>
> —Kareem Abdul-Jabbar

Kareem isn't the only great athlete who's benefited from Hatha Yoga under my teaching—far from it. Tennis legend John McEnroe was also experiencing some physical problems that had forced him to retire from tennis. He came to me and once again, yoga gave him six more years on the court. As his and Kareem's stories show, it's not too late (it's never too late, remember?) to place the smarter bet. No matter how you've been abusing your body, you can repair the damage by switching to the right kind of exercise, applying the right kind of treatment.

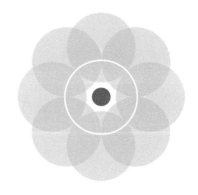

CHAPTER THREE

Bitter Truths: Why America Needs Yoga Now More than Ever

THERE'S A WIDESPREAD SPIRITUAL CRISIS IN THE UNITED States, the country that's embraced me, and the country that I love. The solution is so simple, and I see it so clearly. You guessed it: The solution is yoga. But what I also see clearly is that so many people in today's America are not ready to accept what yoga is offering them, much less take the necessary steps to become a healthy person and a spiritual human being.

In my life I have traveled all over the world, and I chose to live here in America because I wanted to live in the best country on Earth. I've been here for over 35 years now; I am proud and lucky to be able to call myself an American. At the same time, I will always be Indian in my heart. Knowing and loving American people as I do, and seeing you from my Indian perspective, has made me acutely aware that many of you are suffering, and suffering needlessly. It is my mission in life to try to help you out of this unnecessary agony. To do that, I have to push you to change your life—and ultimately, save your life.

Understand that when I say something to "you" in this book, I'm not only talking about just you personally. I am also referring to the collective "you," the hundreds of millions of people in the United States and the billions in the Western world. Since you and I probably haven't met, I don't know whether you are suffering from any of the problems I describe. Maybe your spiritual life and contentment level are already A+—good for you. But you can still come to understand yoga better, improve your practice and your life, and become even happier! As in my classes, my aim in this book is to offer something for everyone. If a problem I describe is not one you are currently experiencing, then the advice can work as preventive medicine, keeping you from possibly going down a wrong path. You will know deep down what applies to you and your circumstances. Take to heart the parts of my advice that you know you need.

Some of it may be difficult for you to hear. Remember, I told you my love was going to be a tough love. As your teacher it's my responsibility to tell you the truth as I see it. Some of the things I'm about to say might make you angry, resentful or defensive. But telling the truth is the only way I know how to help you through the cultural and spiritual challenges you face. In the West, from what I've seen, you are conditioned to believe that when somebody tells you the truth they are insulting you. To avoid offending others, you are taught to say anything in order to make them happy. That means sugarcoating the truth.

But I don't do that. In India, honesty is a requirement of our culture. There, everyone will zero in on your weaknesses and jab them with a needle. Telling you what your problems are is seen as a sign of affection or positive interest, not an insult. What's more, in my life's work, teaching yoga, I have to express myself honestly and effectively to other people, pin-pointing their problems or mistakes in order to help them progress. I don't tell them what they want to hear and I don't sugarcoat—if I did, I wouldn't be Bikram!

In many ways my toughness and truth-telling have been the keys to my success here. If students are late to class by two minutes, I warn them. If they're late again, I throw them out. No excuses. Nobody talks back. It doesn't matter who you are—a famous person, a rich person—nobody breaks the rules. That's part of the discipline, the dignity we learn in yoga. But along with all the toughness, I offer my students my love; they know I just want what's best for them.

In India, our problems are mostly external. For centuries we have suffered from civil wars, religious wars, starvation, overpopulation, oppression, drought and flood. My people have survived these trials by evolving a highly developed system for finding happiness and contentment within. Many times I have brought Westerners to India for the first time and their reaction is always the same. "Everyone is so happy here! How is this possible?" The answer is that my people came to see that only inner peace lasts, and only Self-Realization rewards the human spirit. All else is meaningless.

Here in the West, you are materially blessed; your outer world is one of comfort and beauty. There is no excuse for suffering! Of course, not everyone is rich in this richest country on Earth, or even comfortable. But if you've chosen to buy this book I would imagine that you have enough money to eat and a decent place in which to live, that you have some degree of ease. You probably have a good job, a nice car, a nice house, maybe some sweet kids and a loving spouse. Still, you may be unhappy. Even if you don't have any major problems, you may simply have an uneasy feeling that something is missing, or a yearning for something you can't put your finger on. Why?

To a large degree, your problems are internal: You suffer from anger, greed, insecurity, a sense of entitlement, depression, disconnection, corruption and loneliness. The outward manifestation of these problems is crime, divorce, pollution, child abuse, drug and alcohol abuse. Our children are simultaneously spoiled and neglected; the elderly are left in isolation. Too many Americans' bodies wind up as broken as their marriage vows, and the closer they come to death, the more they fear it. They can't bear to face their problems head-on, so instead they major in avoidance and denial.

Don't like the way your day is going? Why not just have a drink or a smoke or take a pill, legal or otherwise, and forget about your troubles for a while? So what if the problems are still there when you wake up? You'll just go out looking for new and improved ways to run and hide from your life. These are all cultural problems, not individual ones. You deserve better information, better guidance: You need the Eastern philosophy of life. But you're not getting it.

In India we have a Hindi saying: *"Aram haram, hai."* *Aram* means "comfort;" *haram* means "to destroy;" and *hai* means "ease." "Comfort destroys ease." This is a fairly new phenomenon. Thousands of years ago, if you were able to take shelter with your family in a tiny cave without freezing to death or being eaten by a saber-toothed tiger, you were happy. If you could spend all day out in the cold hunting for food, return home with a rabbit, burn your food over an open fire and eat it, you would have a peaceful sleep. That's why I say the biggest problem in life is *no problem*—not having to occupy your mind with survival. As Americans are finding out, having big, shiny bathrooms and designer clothes, or building stadiums, freeways and sleek office towers, does not create happiness—in fact, it destroys it.

Another way of saying this is that you have too many choices. In India, most people don't have choices, so they can't get spoiled, or take the wrong roads. When you have no choice—like when your guru or spiritual master tells you to do something—the only way is obviously the right way, and the right way is the hard way. That's what we do in my yoga classes; we give you no choice. You have to do it the right way. The whole class is one big brainwashing session—washing out bad habits and old patterns that keep you from experienceing mental peace, happiness, and a satisfaction in living.

Now that I live in America and I'm successful, I have too many choices, too. In the morning I stand in front of my closet wondering which shirt I should wear. Which pants? Which shoes will match? I have too many choices. Once I am dressed I go to the board where I hang all my car keys and try to decide which of my cars to drive. Do you believe it?

Without the philosophy of Vedanta Yoga, you have no higher purpose in your life, no final destination on your journey. As we say in India, you're spitting at the sky. (In America, you say pissing in the wind.) Without a solid grounding in yoga, you have not yet learned to master your ego-controlled mind. As a result, you create mental problems for yourself. One of the worst of those problems is anger. So many people are so angry, and this is true all over the world. If the traffic is a little slow, they get mad. Somebody cuts in front of them in line, they get into a fight. They hold grudges, and families feud. You've seen this, right?

If there is no moderation within your mind, no balance of biochemistry through the sustained practice of yoga, every fraction of a second you are disturbed by something or somebody around you. Anything can make you fly off the handle or spiral down into the abyss of depression. The physical symptoms of this mental imbalance are a grim checklist of the most common American ailments: depression, heart disease, high blood pressure, diabetes, cancer, gastrointestinal disorders, obesity.

Psychiatrists in the United States write millions of prescriptions for Prozac and other psychoactive drugs every year. Do you need these? No! All they do is put the brain to sleep, put you in a waking coma; they don't solve the problem.

You've created this cultural mess and it's up to you to fix it. As we say in India, if you dig a canal and invite a crocodile into your bedroom, don't blame the crocodile when he bites your ass! Is everything and everybody really so great in India? Of course not! I've just told you some of the terrible problems we have there, not the least of which is trying to feed more than a billion people. And we practically invented the concept of discrimination with the caste system, which is a terrible thing. But we are survivors, and to deal with our problems, we've developed a system that lets us find peace within no matter what the conditions around us. In India it is said that when a yogi is meditating, an atom bomb detonating could not distract him. Instead, the yogi would swallow the explosion and digest it. That is the power of yoga and the power of yogis.

In so much of the world today, connection is the missing ingredient. Why do people fight and divorce? Lack of connection, mutual understanding, and real communication. Too many of us live in isolation, disconnected from each other and the Earth we share with the rest of humanity. The countries of the world are increasingly isolated from one another. But yoga and the traditions of the East recognize that union—true connection—is vital for a satisfying and rewarding life.

Come on, wake up. You've been sleeping too long. You're not living the right way, not satisfied? It's okay. Our ancient land of India has a long tradition of gurus, great teachers handing down spiritual wisdom. Let us help you end your anger and your mental and emotional imbalances. It can be done. You can live better lives than anyone else on the planet. You know why I say that?

Because of all the great things about America and Americans. You are uniquely gifted, and uniquely positioned, to integrate the best the East has to offer with the best of the West. You can do it because you're innovators; you embrace change. Every day you discover new ways to succeed, and you have taught me so much about creativity, organization and success. In India some of our great traditions have held us back. Though this is not as true as it once was, in the past we have been very old-fashioned, stubborn and afraid of new ideas. Up until very recently, we would rather waste talent than break with tradition. We were backward-thinking where you are forward-thinking. America has innovated more in the last 200 years than the rest of the world put together. Your contributions to the worlds of science and industry, art and entertainment have benefited everyone. What's right is what works, and you have clearly done a lot right here.

Though I love all of humanity, I particularly love Americans because it is so easy to communicate with you. You are very open-hearted and open-minded. On top of that, you are smart. You invite people from other cultures to share their spiritual wisdom: Gandhi, the Dalai Lama, Swami Vivekenanda, Paramahansa Yogananda. That wonderful quality is why so many successful people here will spend time and money listening to some bigmouth from the streets of Calcutta tell them what to do, even tell them some things that they really don't want to hear.

I believe that you have reached the stage as a country and as individuals where you can finally make your minds your best friends. When you can finally wake up. It's not time to smell the coffee, it's time to change. All you need are the right tools, the right keys. You can't start a Cadillac with a Toyota key; yoga is the master key that opens all doors.

Add the spiritual, traditional Eastern way of yoga to the resourceful, inventive American way, and you can have a better life. Remember: It's all about union and it's all about balance. In this marriage of the Eastern and Western approaches to life, you'll achieve a balance of the internal and the external, the mental and the physical, the spiritual and the material. In creating and embodying this new union, you can have—and realize—the best of both worlds. Combine inner peace with outer success. Live the best life possible, the best life ever imagined. That's what I want for you.

We don't have to give up anything; we just need to add to our lives that which is missing. We are only limited by our imaginations, our thoughts and dreams. Everything is attainable with enough hard work. I've done it, and so can you. I'm Indian, but

America is where I found the best life. My Indian homeland never even knew how to provide a public bathroom. (When my student, Mrs. Indira Gandhi, asked me what should be done to serve the people of India, I said, "Build some public restrooms so people don't have to piss in the streets like dogs.") You follow me? I benefit from the land of yogis and ancient wisdom as well as from America, the unrivaled land of opportunity. I consider it the perfect balance, and I never take the life I created for granted.

I've been hammering you about all your problems, what you and your culture lack, but let's turn that around, and see the positive possibilities—the good news. If you lack Spirituality, who will profit most from being exposed to it? *You* will! And because it's new to you and you're not yet tired of hearing it, you can also absorb this message better. This book offers you the opportunity to read, sit, think, and ultimately to take a U-turn on the ride of your life. I'm not just going to criticize and tell you your problems—I will also give you the solutions. There's good news along with the bad news, and I'll tell you both. I will make a yogi, a truly spiritual human being, out of you yet.

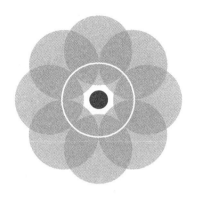

CHAPTER FOUR

Right Road, Wrong Direction: How American Yoga Lost Its Way

The theory advanced by certain ignorant writers that yoga is "unsuitable for Westerners" is wholly false, and has lamentably prevented many sincere students from seeking its manifold blessings. Yoga cannot know a barrier of East and West any more than does the healing and equitable light of the sun.

—Paramahansa Yogananda

"BUT BIKRAM," I CAN HEAR YOU SAYING, "WHY DO YOU KEEP yelling at us that we need to do yoga? We *are* doing yoga! You of all people should know how popular yoga's become in the United

States in the past 10 years or so. Maybe *you* need to wake up, open *your* eyes, and realize we've already taken your advice. What's your problem?"

Of course, my friends, I know that yoga is now trendy, popular and a subject for glossy magazine covers; I even read somewhere over 20 million people in the United States say they practice yoga. And that's a big number. But numbers can lie. To explain, I will ask *you* a question: What kind of yoga are all those people doing? Bogus yoga, that's what kind. *That's* my problem, and your problem. It's an obstacle that continues to block the liberation of the West, individually and collectively. It's the next speed bump you have to pass on your drive to the perfect life, and it's a big one.

Lucky for you, you are about to experience the solution: my pure yoga Sequence of 26 postures and two breathing exercises. Let me now explain why you can only reach the goals we've been discussing by practicing my Bikram Yoga, and not some infomercial junk yoga. To understand why so many of those millions of students—and up until now, you may have been one of them—aren't getting what they paid for, but rather a bill of knockoff goods, I need to educate you about your own history, a part of America's past that most citizens are completely unaware of. I'm talking about how yoga came to America.

Swami Vivekenanda was the first Indian spiritual master to visit the modern West. He came to the United States in September 1893 (when he was 27) to speak at the World Parliament of Religions, part of the Columbian Exposition in Chicago. His speech on Vedanta and Raja Yoga was so well received that he was subsequently booked for a lecture tour throughout the United States. When he left America, Vivekenanda told people that another yogi would follow him, and named as his successor Swami Paramahansa Yogananda, my guru's older brother. Remarkably, at the time of Swami Vivekenanda's prophecy, Paramahansa Yogananda was less than one year old.

The famed author of *Autobiography of a Yogi*, Paramahansa Yogananda, came to Boston in 1920 and stayed there five years, teaching the eight limbs of yoga according to Patanjali's Yoga Sutras. In addition, he taught his disciples an advanced yogic breathing and meditation technique that he called Kriya Yoga, "the airplane route to God." In 1924, Yogananda went on a spiritual campaign across the United States, spreading the message of Self-Realization. Hundreds of thousands of Americans filled lecture halls to hear the great Indian swami's impassioned speeches. In 1925 he established the International Headquarters of the Self-Realization Fellowship in Glendale, California.

In the early 1930s, Yogananda and his youngest brother, Bishnu Ghosh, traveled together throughout the United States giving lectures and demonstrations of physical culture including bodybuilding and Hatha Yoga. At Yogananda's request, my guru also started teaching Hatha Yoga at the Self-Realization Fellowship. Ghosh inspired both children and adults to strengthen their bodies and minds. My guru also originated bodybuilding contests in America, founding the Mr. Universe contest and acting as its chief judge in 1948. He was an Olympic judge, a member of the International Olympic Committee, and founder of the International Weightlifting and Body Building Federation. He also became a visiting professor at Columbia University, though he continued to return to India often in order to train yogis at his own school, Ghosh's College of Physical Education, in Calcutta.

Following my guru and his son-in-law, Buddha Bose, three more significant yogis came to the United States. The first to arrive was Bishnu Devananda, who was followed by Swami Satchitananda. They were both disciples of Swami Sivananda and considered powerful yogis. Then, in the early 1970s, B. K. S. Iyengar, a yogi from Pune, near Bombay, arrived. Unfortunately, these three yogis and others felt that the American people and their bodies were just not capable of practicing real, traditional Indian yoga. They responded by changing the true yoga they'd been taught into something they thought Americans could more readily accomplish and understand. Frankly, they didn't think you could handle the truth.

What did they do because of their lack of faith in Western people and the sacred teaching of their gurus? How did they screw up their sacred duty? First, they changed some of Patanjali's original 84 postures to accommodate the inflexibility of American bodies, and stopped teaching other postures they thought would be too hard. Another of the worst bastardizations was that they loosened or abandoned the rigorous discipline with which yoga must be taught, the way they themselves came to be yoga masters. Americans, they mistakenly believed, should not be pushed out of their "comfort zone." Next came all the bizarre props, including ropes, straps, chairs, pulleys, benches, whips, chains, clamps and other unnecessary crutches to try to help Western bodies get into the postures. Iyengar uses so many props in his method that he's called "The Furniture Yogi" in India. All of this compromised the true way and diluted Hatha Yoga.

This dilution that these yogis caused was passed down to their disciples and then to their well-meaning American students who became teachers themselves. These American teachers then proceeded to take yoga even further in the wrong direction. We all know that Americans are highly inventive; there's a Thomas Edison around every corner here. Sure enough, American yoga teachers invented posture after posture, modification after modification, making up their own Sanskrit names, and then selling their defective wares to the uninitiated. Now you find, to list just a few, things like Kundalini Yoga and Ashtanga Yoga, which never existed in India. Kundalini refers to the energy channel that runs between all the chakras or energy centers in the body. The name Ashtanga is derived from the Sanskrit word *ashta*, meaning "eight"; it refers to the eight limbs of yoga or the Eight-fold Path. But these things (and so-called Vinyasa Yoga) are not part of the original yoga; there is only Hatha. Bikram Yoga is Hatha Yoga.

These days, the yoga "brands" are getting even more ridiculous; you've got Easy Yoga, Sit-at-Your-Desk Yoga, Yoga for Beginners, Yoga for Dummies, Yoga for Pets, and Babaar Yoga. It's all Mickey Mouse Yoga to me. I don't want to be too harsh; I know these teachers are sincere, and if they are trying in their own ways to promote yoga, there's good in that. It's just that many of these invented methods have eliminated some of the most essential and beneficial elements of yoga, its very heart and soul! Students here often aren't taught to freeze the body in the postures for the prescribed number of seconds. Some teachers ignore the fact that you must maintain proper control of the breath in each posture, and that proper breathing varies according to individual postures. And almost all yoga taught here today fails to give you enough time in *Savasana*, the "Dead Body Pose," or posture of complete relaxation. Some have turned yoga into just a fitness activity, one that doesn't give you the true physical or Spiritual benefit. Maybe some calisthenic benefit, that's all.

These improper teachings can be downright dangerous; I can't tell you how many people come to my class to heal injuries they've incurred through the practice of diluted Hatha Yoga. I agree that not everyone must perform all 84 original postures; that's why I invented my Sequence of 26 postures and two breathing exercises. But the postures you do *must* be actual yoga *asanas*, and not something created out of thin air. That is not yoga. Yogurt maybe, but not yoga, and it won't give anyone yoga's therapeutic benefits.

After some of these well-meaning but misguided knockoff artists preceded me, you can imagine that when I got here 40 years ago and tried to teach yoga the way my guru taught me, people looked at me as if I were from another planet. But with English bulldog determination I remained steadfast in my methods, believing that the people of the Western world could only fully benefit from trying things *the right way*. This system has worked in India for thousands of years, and it will work for the rest of the world because underneath it all, we are the same. I would not have been able to look at myself in the mirror if I had compromised the great tradition I was chosen to represent. For me, teaching yoga the right way was the only choice.

If some things are too hard for the students, for their weak bodies, then I make it harder! This is the only way for human beings to break free from their self-imposed limitations and begin to understand that *there are no limitations*. I believed in the strength of the Western people and decided it was simply a matter of teaching discipline through the postures in order to reach them.

It wasn't easy. I was shocked to see how many Americans came to class late, drank water at the slightest hint of thirst, complained about the heat—you name it. At first, when my students didn't get their way, they got mad at me. But while they were always free to leave, most never did. Their experience in Bikram's Torture Chamber made them realize they could overcome any obstacles in spite of the "hardships" I imposed in class. This was a revelation to them, one I want to share with you: *They had power they didn't even know they had.* And when they realized it, they were able to carry that power with them out of the studio and into their everyday lives.

All you need is to be shown a better way, the true way of Hatha Yoga. It's like this: If you've only seen a car driven in Reverse, you will never understand that the faster, safer way to get somewhere is to put it in Drive. Once you understand that, you can move forward. (And you'll stop getting a stiff neck from craning around to look behind you when you're at the wheel!)

Let me encourage you the way I encourage all my students. Can't do a particular yoga posture today? If you persist in trying the right way, a day will come when you can. Don't cheat or change the posture to conform to your individual weaknesses. If you do, the real benefit goes out the window. Would you rather suffer for 90 minutes or 90 years? The right way is the hard way, and it's up to you to make it work. Remember: *"It's never too late, it's never too bad, and you're never too old or too sick to start from scratch once again."*

PART TWO

The Bikram Yoga Practice

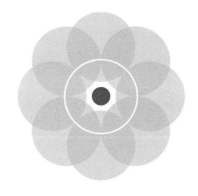

CHAPTER FIVE

How Yoga Works: The Science of My Sequence

I'M OFTEN ASKED HOW I CAME UP WITH MY UNIQUE SEQUENCE of 26 postures and two breathing exercises. You remember that I first started developing it in India in order to treat many people at once, rather than administering different *asanas* and *pranayamas* to each patient of Bishnu Ghosh. By working as his assistant I learned through hands-on experience the therapeutic value of every aspect of Hatha Yoga for various common health problems. Of course by that time I knew the original 84 postures he'd taught me inside and out; through my practice I'd been researching the effects of yoga in the laboratory of my own body. That also helped me to understand what would work for others.

From there I calculated that it took these specific 26 postures to systematically work every part of the body, to give all the internal organs, all the veins, all the ligaments, and all the muscles everything they need to maintain optimum health and maximum function. Although I teach the traditional 84-posture practice in its entirety to my teachers and most advanced students in Los Angeles, they all continue to learn and benefit from my Sequence, also known as the "beginning series." Each component takes care of something different in the body, and yet they all work together synergistically, contributing to the success of every other one, and extending its benefits.

The structure of the Sequence is 90 percent science, 10 percent inspiration. You'll see, for example, that as we get further into the class and the body is warmer and more limber, we perform the postures that call for deeper stretching and bending. If you start right off with the Spine Twisting posture, I guarantee you will not receive any benefits; in fact, you'll probably injure your spine. As we progress in the Sequence we will also hone your concentration to its highest level in the last part of the class—before you can go deeply within, your mind has to be prepared and warmed up, too.

Doing two sets, or repetitions, of each posture was also based on my practice and observations: In the first set you explore, you see where you are today. The second time, you go deeper, with more confidence. You attack the posture and you nail it! Remember, even though I call this a beginning series, it will be challenging for everyone, regardless of their experience level.

So the Sequence is logical, practical and scientific. At the same time, though, there was something very intuitive about the way I invented it. That's the inspiration part. I think of it this way: With the 26 letters in the English alphabet you can create millions of different words, and through them, any meaning you want. Your words can inspire people, build civilizations, create beauty and even end wars. In music you can create millions of melodies with just eight notes. Music can also inspire people or move them to tears. In both cases it all depends on how you arrange those building blocks, or component parts.

Millions of books, millions of melodies. Like all the great writers and composers, I, too, benefited from divine inspiration in the creation of my art. I believed there was a beautiful song that the body could sing to the soul, so I attempted to write it. That song, as I heard it, is the Sequence. That's the best answer I can give.

Bikram Yoga 101: The Basics

To continue your introduction to Bikram Yoga, I'd like to answer some more of the questions my beginning students—and even the experienced ones—often ask. You've seen the term FAQ, meaning Frequently Asked Questions? Well, these are BFAQ— Bikram's Frequently Asked Questions, with much more complete and specific answers than I am able to give in person to my classes. Hey, we only have 90 minutes in there. I can't stand around explaining all day!

For sure, the most common question I get is *"Why is it so damn hot in here?!?!?!"*

Walk into one of my classrooms and the first thing you will feel is that it's hot. Very hot. Ideally, each one of Bikram's Torture Chambers is heated to 105 degrees. Why? Think of the blacksmith. If he wants to hammer a hunk of metal into a beautiful sword, the first thing he has to do is put it in the fire. When the iron is glowing red and completely soft, he brings it out and slowly starts hammering it and shaping it into a strong, resilient, razor-sharp blade.

It's the same with yoga. Yoga changes the construction of the body from the inside out, from bones to skin and from fingertips to toes. So before you change it, you have to heat it up to soften it, because a warm body is a flexible body. Then you can reshape the body any way you want.

At first it will probably feel too hot. You may want to run out of the room to get some cool air. Of course, I won't let you. The right way is the hard way! After six months you will only notice the heat if the room isn't hot *enough*. Remember, yoga was developed in India, where every room is hot. In order to mimic Indian heat in the chilly West, especially for people who have never touched their toes or done a backward bend in their lives, we have to turn up the thermostat. The heat will initially serve to allow you to twist and stretch with less chance of injury. (Yes, some people get hurt in yoga classes, even mine. Most injuries occur when the students overdo it, trying to accomplish too much too soon, or don't follow the instructions they're given. But overall, yoga is extremely safe if done correctly.) Eventually, you learn to generate your own heat and come to rely on it less for injury prevention than as a tool for enhancing flexibility and deepening an awareness of breath.

You may have seen that some in the so-called medical community have criticized my method, declaring, "Doing exercise in

a hot room is bad for high blood pressure and bad for the heart."
They also claim that it's bad for people with multiple sclerosis,
hepatitis C, and high cholesterol. Well, I have been practicing
and teaching Hatha Yoga this way for more than 50 years. If what
these critics say is true, hundreds of thousands of people who had
these kinds of maladies should be *dead* from taking my class. But
they're not. Instead, they get better, often making remarkable
recoveries. What's right is what works, so it follows that I am
actually doing a better job than most specialists and cardiologists—
Western allopathic doctors—are doing. Maybe that's why they
don't like me, those fakers. Don't get me started on them. Let's
move on to the next question.

"Bikram, why is there no meditation in your classes?"

But there is, my friend.

"Which part?"

All of it! My yoga class is taught as a 90-minute meditation,
combining Hatha and Raja Yoga—and you can bet you're performing some concentrated Karma Yoga as well. If you don't see
how something so physically demanding can be called a meditation, consider this.

Let's say there's a special room in your house just for meditation. Everything about it is conducive to peaceful contemplation, and you can walk in, lock the door, take the phone off the
hook and be completely undisturbed anytime you want. You sit
down on your favorite soft meditation pillow, light your favorite
incense, play your favorite relaxing music, and begin your meditation. Great. Enjoy. You know what you're going to get from
this kind of meditation? A fat ass and a lazy body.

Now, imagine that you are stuck in rush-hour traffic in the
middle of the summer. It's about 102 degrees outside, your air-
conditioning is broken and your window rolls down only half-

way. You're 45 minutes late for the most important meeting of your life, the same wonderful human being in the blue van just cut you off for the third time, and you really have to pee. Now, if you can find peace *under those conditions*, then you can meditate anywhere.

My yoga class is that sweltering day. It's one long, hot meditation. We put incredible pressure on you to teach you to break your attachment to external things and go within. Instead of blaming others for your own weakness, fear and depression, you will learn to take responsibility for your own life. You've got to face yourself in the mirror, every part you don't like, every mistake you make, every excuse your mind creates to limit your potential liberation—there's nowhere to run, nowhere to hide. No escape from reality. With these kinds of demands on your abilities and attention, you will soon forget that there is anyone on the next mat in the classroom, much less notice what they are wearing. After you learn to discipline your body and mind under these conditions, you will truly be able to concentrate; no external will be able to break your powerful focus. That's why I say that the darkest place in the world is under the brightest lamp. In the Torture Chamber of my class, you will find a beautiful light, and the source of that light is within you.

"Why meditate anyway? What does meditation actually mean?"

Meditation is the practice of focusing and calming the mind in order to communicate with the God inside you, your Self or Spirit, eventually leading to true communion with your Spirit, or Self-Realization. Called *Puja* in India, meditation traditionally requires sitting alone in a room, on a boat, in a temple, under a tree, or wherever, and concentrating your mind on one thing for a long time while keeping it free from all the countless distractions of this world.

In attempting to focus your attention, you need something to concentrate on or think about. What should you choose? Well, if you listen to the religious stories, God says, "Think about me." If you were inclined to choose Lord Krishna as your representation of God, you might say "Hare Krishna, Hare Krishna, Krishna, Krishna, Hare, Hare, Hare Rama, Hare Rama, Rama, Rama, Hare, Hare . . ." over and over again as a mantra. Or you can say the Lord's Prayer. Mantras are sounds, words or groups of words that can be uttered repetitively and rhythmically to induce a meditative state. Chant the mantra and you won't be distracted by anything else.

My guru gave me my mantra, and I still use it every day and try to make it a part of me every fraction of every second of my life. I'm very proud of my mantra, and though I'm not supposed to reveal it, I think it's okay; I want to share the idea of this very powerful tool with you. Translated from Sanskrit, it means *Serve your Self; you are born to give, not to get.* We believe that giving to others is the best way to serve the Self; that's how I fulfill my Karma Yoga, or sacred duty, by helping you, and by so doing I am realized and fulfilled.

If you want to attempt more meditation on your own, outside of my studio, using the traditional sitting methods and even a mantra, that's fine. It's probably a good idea. As your Hatha yoga teacher, though, I am more concerned with the physical plane. That's where yoga begins. My job is to help you to prepare your body, which will quiet the mind, and begin to build a solid foundation for a Spiritual life. Though I will discuss Spiritual matters at length in this book, it all comes back to one basic principle: Practice your yoga!

"Okay, Bikram, how do you *meditate?*"

I meditate when I'm waxing my cars. I meditate when I'm

teaching yoga, when I'm shopping, watching old Hindi movies, driving, dancing, singing, talking, eating and spending time with my kids. I meditate all the time, because my mind is my best friend. I make my life my meditation. I don't think this is the answer most people expect. What can I do?

"Bikram, how often must I practice?"

Well, how often do you plan on using your body? I don't know you that well, but I'm guessing you pretty much use it daily. Even when you are sitting there watching TV or sleeping, your body is working to keep you alive. As they function, the cells, the glands and the organs all create waste products, toxins. Even the organs that eliminate waste create waste. So once every day you must flush out each and every gland and organ. You need to clean your body from the inside out, just like you eat, like you sleep, like you brush your teeth or shower.

Hatha Yoga flushes away the waste products, the toxins of all the glands and organs of your body. It provides a natural irrigation of the body through the circulatory system, with the help of the respiratory system. It brings nourishment to every cell of your body so that each one can perform its function and keep your body healthy. My yoga system also employs heat to further that cleansing process: When you sweat, impurities are flushed out of the body through the skin. And you *will* sweat, believe me.

So you must practice your Hatha Yoga every day. If you don't, your body will break down like a car that isn't maintained properly.

How Yoga Heals

Like my Sequence, Hatha Yoga works in many complex ways. I'll explain some of those ways here, then tell you more as we actually go through the Sequence, including the specific medical benefits of each posture and how yoga combats various diseases and imbalances, from diabetes to stress to obesity.

The essential qualities of a healthy body are strength and flexibility and maintaining the proper balance between those two things. No human being is born with strength and flexibility balanced correctly. The best ballerina in the world can't hold a Hatha Yoga balancing posture longer than three seconds. Like most flexible people's muscles, hers don't have enough strength. So in yoga we first use what we are born with to get what we need. If you are strong, use that strength to develop flexibility. If you were born with flexibility, use it to increase your strength. When your strength and flexibility are at the same level, you don't have to try to balance—the body will balance itself. Once you have a perfectly healthy body, then you have to balance it with the mind.

Another overall way yoga heals is by serving as a diagnostic tool. Your inability to hold a posture correctly can often tell you which parts of your body are weak or not functioning well. Like a good mechanic, you'll be running a diagnostic checkup on yourself, locating imbalances to be worked on and organs or other systems in need of repair. Here are some of the most important entries on that checklist, specific ways that yoga heals the different components of the human body.

Breathing and the Lungs

Improving the function of the lungs is almost always the first repair that needs doing. That's why the first thing we practice is *pranayama*, a breathing exercise that increases your puny lung capacity. Don't feel bad; you and your lungs shouldn't take that personally. Most people spend their entire lives rarely using more than 50 percent of their total lung capacity. In the beginning your lungs will feel tight and small, which is perfectly normal. With each additional class, you will find that your breath becomes deeper and fuller. Your lungs are like balloons—they must be properly inflated and stretched to become more flexible and capable of holding and processing more oxygen with greater efficiency.

The lungs are a high-powered purification plant, separating environmental pollutants from the essential oxygen in the air. If the lungs failed to filter out carbon monoxide, for example, death would result almost immediately. When the lungs do their job, they send fresh oxygen throughout the body, purifying the blood and allowing it to travel more efficiently via the arteries and the heart. But when the lungs aren't functioning optimally, they're unable to keep up, to constantly purify 100 percent of the supplied air. Maybe they are only capable of purifying 40 percent of the air supply, leaving a full 60 percent unfiltered. To add further insult to injury, you may even insist upon smoking cigarettes! At this stage, your immune system goes into a veritable coma, paralyzing your defenses. This creates all sorts of problems such as asthma, bronchitis, and emphysema and even accelerates the aging process.

That's right: People are aging much faster than they should because of this slow death by oxygen deprivation. Doctors don't know how to help people breathe properly to prevent disease. They do their limited best by providing medication, but that's not nearly enough. Only the yogis know this. Proper breathing and control of the breath are parts of the yogic discipline and have been for thousands of years.

Breath is life. This lesson was brought home to me with great force back in 1971, when I was teaching in Tokyo. One Sunday night I was just about to go out (to the movies, of course) when the phone rang. I was summoned to the Israeli Embassy, in the section of town called Budokan; a woman named Ursula Battur, who was the wife of the Israeli ambassador, was dying of cancer. Her husband called for me in a desperate attempt to prolong her life.

She could only breathe through an oxygen mask, which covered her face as I entered her bedroom. The room was full of friends and relatives, as well as a rabbi. They believed she only had hours to live, so they had assembled to begin mourning her. The first thing I did was clear the room. "Everybody out!" I yelled. "Get out of here!" Some of the people there weren't too happy with me at that point, especially the rabbi.

But I threw them all out and opened the window. I remember that it had just started snowing outside, and the flakes started drifting in through the window. Then I went over to her bed and got her to sit up, propping her up on some pillows. I took the oxygen mask off and said, "Ursula, if you understand what I'm saying, smile." I can still see the smile warming her face, and feel my guru's power and confidence coursing through my veins. It gave me goose bumps and made my hair stand on end. I transferred his cosmic power from my body to Ursula's. I sat down on the bed in front of her and led her through some deep inhaling and exhaling. I did this *pranayama* breathing with her from about

6 p.m. to midnight, when she got up, went to the bathroom and drank some water—she even ate some leftover food from the gathering they had called to observe her death.

I went to the Embassy three times a week for eight months, teaching her yoga. A little while later, Mr. Battur became finance minister of Israel, so they had to move back to Tel Aviv. Then I received a message that Ursula had passed away—one year and eight months after she was supposed to. Everybody thought I had performed magic in that room. No! I just showed her how to breathe again, clearing her trachea. *Pranayama* saved her life— not magic, and certainly not me.

A few years later, I was teaching in Waikiki Beach in Hawaii, working with an organization called YPO, the Young Presidents Organization, which includes many of the richest and most important people in the world under 40. I met an Israeli man who told me he was eager to come to my class at 6 the next morning, adding, "I have great respect for yoga teachers." I asked him why—and he proceeded to tell me the whole story of Ursula Battur, and how some yoga teacher had saved her life in Japan!

"Sir," I finally told him, "I am that yoga teacher." Was he in class the next morning? You better believe it.

Heart and Lungs: Respiratory Partners

Most people don't realize that respiratory function is not confined to the lungs. True health requires that the lungs and the heart work well together, as in a happy marriage or a successful business partnership. The heart is like a trucking company under contract to distribute food (blood) to the rest of the body. The lungs run a supplier company, which provides the heart with fuel (oxygen). When business is good, the respiratory system and the circulatory system are a team, working together to deliver fresh, oxygenated blood to every system, internal organ, gland and tissue in the body.

Too often, though, their relationship is dysfunctional and their joint business venture goes bad. Lungs Unlimited wants to know why Heart Co.'s shipments of blood are just sitting around at their depot instead of going out to their shared customers. Heart Co. fires back that it's not receiving the oxygen promised by Lungs Unlimited. The companies send sternly worded e-mails back and forth, then they threaten to sue. And all the while, guess who's really at fault?

You are! Heart Co. and Lungs Unlimited are both wholly owned subsidiaries of You, Inc. You're the owner—they're in your body, after all—and if you're not exercising properly, if you're not practicing Hatha Yoga, you disrupt the supply chain and cripple the whole enterprise. You're responsible for the lungs' inability to ship oxygen to the heart and all the other customers in the body.

If, on the other hand, you *do* exercise by practicing Hatha Yoga, you enhance oxygen conversion and absorption and improve blood circulation. Your lungs are now an ultra-efficient purification plant, capable of filtering 10 pounds of oxygen every minute. Now you can inhale and purify the most polluted air from Mexico City, Hong Kong and Calcutta, if need be. In fact, since you only require one pound of oxygen a minute, Heart Co. and Lungs Unlimited not only break even, but make a huge profit! Good business all around.

Practicing yoga not only increases our supplies of oxygen, but it also teaches us how to *use* that oxygen properly—we learn to control the breath through *pranayama*. Someone who doesn't practice yoga takes in oxygen the way a hungry dog takes in food. When you come home at the end of your workday and finally feed him, he will fall on the food and devour it all in half a second. (The part that doesn't fall out of the bowl and go all over the floor, that is.) Untrained lungs will also suck in all the air they can, as fast as they can. In yoga we learn to sustain the breath, not gasp it all in and out, and that means our whole operation runs more efficiently.

Blood and Circulation

Blood is the transporter of oxygen and also nutrition, in the form of glucose, to every cell. Veins and arteries act as the superhighways of the circulatory system, transporting blood throughout the body. All of the postures in my series work to increase the flow of fresh, oxygenated blood to every part of the body. The key dynamic here is a process I call Extension and Compression. Here's how it works.

When you stretch one part of your body, you stretch out the veins and arteries contained there, and their inside diameter becomes smaller and smaller. The normal amount of blood cannot flow through these narrowed passageways, so the heart starts pumping harder, trying to accomplish what it normally does. That's the extension. Simultaneously, you are compressing different glands and organs as a result of the particular *asana* you are performing. For example, when you are doing Standing Separate Leg Head to Knee Pose, you compress the pancreas, squeezing the blood out of it like a sponge. Remember, the stretching is compressing and tightening the veins outside the organ, cutting off blood flow like a temporary tourniquet.

All the while, the blood driven by the excited heart is approaching the pancreas like a flood. But it can't go in; the flood is blocked because the gates are closed. So outside the pancreas the blood level is rising and rising. It's like the Hoover Dam! Then after 20 seconds in the posture, the blood's volume and pressure have reached maximum capacity, and what do you do? You come out of the pose, open the gates, and blood rushes in and floods the pancreas. Boom! In this way you reenergize, revitalize and clean it in a brief period of time through this one *asana*.

At the same time, this extremely high volume of rich oxygenated blood rushing through your circulatory system is toning the veins and arteries themselves. If there is any kind of bacteria, infection, germ or virus in there, the dynamic internal changes in volume, speed and pressure blow them out. No more arteriosclerosis, no more varicose veins. My yoga series has cured countless students of these afflictions.

No other form of exercise can create this volume and force. Running, for example, can elevate your heart rate, and with each beat, the blood flows. But that blood is being distributed equally all over your body, from top to bottom. That means each organ and system is just getting a tiny taste, a *little* more blood—its "fair share"—not a big increase. Let me give you an illustration from where I live, Los Angeles.

You may know that we have water shortages out here in the West, and someday, if development and population growth don't slow down, it is going to be a big problem. Let's say that day has come. Los Angeles has many cities within it, and if the water department sends them all water at the same time, all anyone gets is a trickle. So the city says, "Every half hour we will supply water to each city in turn. At 6 a.m. we will have water only in the city of Beverly Hills. At 6:30 it will stop and

the water will go to Culver City." And so on. This way, everyone gets more than a trickle and—*ahhh*—they can take a nice
shower. At the appointed time, everyone gets enough water
pressure.

It's all about extension and compression. This is happening in
every phase of yoga, all the time. Every time you bend to the
right, you are compressing or closing that side while opening up
the left side. And vice versa. The moment you release the posture, blood is transported from one side to the other. In this way
you sequentially improve each part of the whole human body.
This process, and the benefits of compression and extension, is
completed when you follow certain postures with *Savasana*,
which I'll explain later.

The Brain

The brain is immersed in cerebrospinal fluid and consists of more
than 100 billion neurons. It represents only 2 or 3 percent of the
body's total weight, but it uses over 20 percent of the body's energy. It relentlessly demands oxygen, glucose and all kinds of nutrients, which it uses to regulate every function of the body. To
supply the hungry brain with all these nutrients requires 25 percent of all the blood pumped by the heart.

The 26-posture Sequence works on several levels to improve
brain function and balance. First, by removing impediments from
the musculoskeletal and circulatory systems, it increases blood
flow, including to the brain. The breathing exercises also greatly
increase the lung's capacity to oxygenate this blood, so the brain
gets more of the fuel it needs. Recent studies conducted at the
Salk Institute of Biological Studies, as well as at Princeton Uni-

versity, confirm that certain kinds of physical and mental exercise not only prolong the life of existing brain cells, but also promote the growth of new neurons in the hippocampus, a part of the brain that plays an important role in maintaining memory. The same thing happens when you do Bikram Yoga: The intense mental concentration required gives the brain a workout, which keeps it strong and sharp well into old age.

The biggest benefit of yoga to the brain is biochemical in nature. Let me explain. In yoga we say there are 11 receiving centers behind each ear that take in sound and other kinds of information—22 in all. And the brain is the central receiving center for all the information we absorb. When we take in negative information—bad news—the brain receives it, identifies it, then sends that bad news out all over the body in the form of biochemical messages. These chemicals are caustic and they produce acids that negatively affect the nerves. (For example, the stress hormones adrenaline and cortisol have long-term damaging effects; see the sidebar on stress in chapter 6.)

But yoga, through the physical movements and the concentration involved, changes that negative brain chemistry, balancing it properly and reducing those caustic acids. In Western medical terms, it decreases the activity of the sympathetic nervous system, also known as your "fight-or-flight response." That's what we do in yoga: We send out millions of good-news messages to our body and brain every second!

The Spine

If you have a strong, healthy spine, the world is yours. My guru used to say: *"The spine is the source of all energy in human life."* It's not just people from the East who know this. Listen to what the great American writer Herman Melville said in *Moby-Dick*:

> *I believe that much of a man's character will be found betokened in his backbone. A thin joist of a spine never yet upheld a full and noble soul. I rejoice in my spine, as in the firm, audacious staff of that flag which I fling half out to the world.*

But if you damage or ruin your spine, your life is over. At best you live in chronic pain; at worst you are a head on a pillow. The spinal column is the most complicated structure in the body; except for the brain and the brain stem, the whole central nervous system passes through it and is protected by its bony structure. In the center of the spine is a passageway for all those nerves; it's filled with spinal fluid, pumped in from the brain. The spinal fluid acts as a shock absorber for the nerves, protecting them from damage. It also provides some nutrition to the nerves and keeps the covering of the nerves soft and pliable. In yogic terms, this cavity is called the *shushumna*, and it's one of the major energy paths in the body.

The spine consists of 24 individual vertebrae connected together, like a bicycle chain, from the coccyx to the occiput, so you have flexibility to bend and twist in every direction. Part of the structure of each vertebra is the foramen, which forms the passageway for nerves and the messages they carry to exit the spinal column and go to the different body parts. For example, in the central part of the spine, the thoracic spine, nerves run to all the glands and organs in the center of the body: the heart, lungs, kidneys, stomach, intestines and so forth.

In sciatica, one of the most common spinal problems, a vertebra at the sacro-lumbar junction of the spine is putting pressure on those nerves. This causes you to feel pain in your hip, legs, feet or other areas, but in fact the pressure is what causes the problem. Since those nerves are meant to serve other important parts of the body, those areas and functions can be compromised as well. And this pain can be excruciating enough to disable an otherwise healthy person.

In this snakelike length of links there's cartilage, hard but pliant. Between every two vertebrae is a disc, a sac of fluid that acts as a shock absorber and provides a cushion to each vertebra. Just like a car's suspension system. Over time, especially if you do some kind of high-impact sports, the repeated shocks from your heel hitting the ground causes narrowing between the vertebrae. (See the sidebar on sports and exercise in chapter 2.) After getting hit over and over with a sledgehammer this way, the springs in your suspension lose some of their strength, and now the two vertebrae hit each other when the spine is impacted, and the cartilage becomes thinner and thinner. As this pressure increases, it compresses the gelatinous material of the disc on one side, causing it to bulge out on the other side, like egg salad getting squeezed out from between the bread in an overstuffed sandwich. This is called a slipped, or herniated, disc.

That bulge can put pressure on the nerves in the spinal cavity, resulting in irritation and swelling. It also decreases the nerve's function, and this condition can worsen until the membrane of the disc ruptures and the gelatinous material in the disc flows into the spinal cavity, changing the delicate chemistry of the spinal fluid.

If you go to a Western doctor, he may fuse the vertebrae, sever the nerves, and take the cartilage out. Though this may decrease the pain, you will essentially be crippled. Or he'll give you some pain pills or anti-inflammatories, which will help a little, until they're yanked from the market in a year or so, when we find out these medicines are actually killing people.

You can still have back trouble even if you don't hurt yourself through exercise. Being sedentary can be just as harmful as being overactive. When they're not used, the muscles of the back become weak and they sag; that, plus the weight of your upper body, causes the spinal column to collapse very slowly. That's one reason old people shrink in height. Medical practitioners think these conditions are normal for people as they age. They don't know that there is a solution to all these problems that has been around for thousands of years.

In yoga we stretch the spine, creating space between the vertebrae, which takes the pressure off the discs. Instead of cutting out vital parts and fusing the remains, yoga *asanas* strengthen and develop the muscles of your back and put you into natural, human traction—instead of mechanical traction—to restore your intervertebral spacing. This way you can keep your spine and the nerves that run through it healthy.

The Intangibles

These are some of the most important ways that yoga acts on the body to create perfect health. Keep in mind, though, that yoga is not reducible to a quantified number of medical benefits. Even as yoga makes measurable changes in your muscles, organs, bones and spine, it also is working on what we call the "subtle anatomy," renewing and reviving you at the cellular level, invisibly taking care of every atom and molecule. There's an emotional and psychological aspect to the healing process as well—the mind/body connection. As much as I like describing things in terms of cars, yoga doesn't just give you a mechanical tune-up. This is soul-stretching we're doing, mind-restoring and Spirit-building. The unquantifiable improvements in your quality of life and your attitude toward life make themselves felt in every cell as well. When you're well, they're well.

One of yoga's most miraculous effects is the way it actually increases your energy, rather than depletes it. After practicing 90 minutes of postures, you're not dragging and exhausted—you're raring to go. Your feet barely touch the ground! How can this be? First, you are in tune, so you operate and process fuel more efficiently. You can go farther on less gas. We also believe that through the breathing exercises, you are generating vastly greater amounts of *prana*, life energy, so naturally you feel more energized. On a medical level, you are taking in more air, oxygenating all your cells and charging them with energy.

My guru quantified this effect; he taught me that one complete Hatha Yoga session infuses the body with enough energy for up to 16 days of health and increased longevity. Practice again the next day and you gain another 16 days, while using only one. It's like putting money in the bank for future use. Put that money in the bank every day, and watch it add up, *with interest.*

I believe it's this energetic surplus that keeps yogis so young. If you're around as many longtime practitioners as I am, you can see that yoga is a regular fountain of youth! When I was teaching in Honolulu, a 93-year-old man used to come to my class every morning at 7 o'clock. He looked like he was 55, maybe 60. He was living the good life, well into old age. People who practice Hatha Yoga seem almost ageless; even the oldest Grandmother Yogini or Grandfather Yogi may appear to be 35 or 40.

Plus, as you age—on the calendar, that is—your yoga practice will only get better. Your capabilities will continue to increase, and your performance will improve, the complete opposite to what occurs through the repetition of almost any other physical activity as you grow older. Don't just take my word for it. The next time you go to class, take some time to observe the veteran practitioners and see for yourself. Good luck keeping up with them, too.

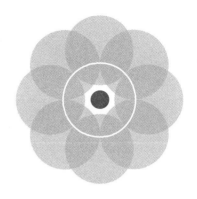

CHAPTER SIX

First Breathing Exercise
Postures 1-4

Plus: Yoga for Stress

THERE ARE THREE ESSENTIAL COMPONENTS OF A TRUE HATHA

Yoga practice:

1. Maintaining relative stillness during the postures

2. Mindful breathing throughout the practice

3. The regular and liberal use of *Savasana*, or Dead Body

    Pose

Without them, you may receive some benefit from yoga, similar to what you would get from calisthenics. You *are* exercising. But you will never receive the 100 percent yoga benefit.

So remember that when you reach your fullest extension in all of these postures—as far as you can go on a given day—you must stay stock-still, holding the position for 10 full seconds or 20, or however long the instruction calls for. Like a statue. Then you'll relax, allowing the blood to circulate and normalize, then you'll stretch again. This alternation, stretching and then relaxing, is where the benefit is. So don't advance and retreat like a nervous puppy. Freeze like a pointer. Students often ask me how they can keep track of the time, or measure how many seconds they've been in a pose. Some try to count their inhalations and exhalations, but breathing patterns vary so much in different people that I recommend beginners place a clock in their line of vision until they get a good sense of how long 10 or 20 seconds feels like, and then they can go back and time it internally.

The second element bears some more explanation, especially for those of you who haven't taken my classes before. For most of the postures I tell you to breathe normally: As you begin to move into each position, inhale as fully as possible, trying to fill the lungs 100 percent, then exhale the breath completely when you achieve the posture. Continue inhaling and exhaling fully while maintaining the posture—this is Normal Breathing, and we'll use this technique during most of the *asanas*.

In a few postures, however, I will call for "80/20 Breathing." (If no technique is specified, use Normal Breathing.) To do this, you inhale fully—whatever 100 percent is for you—but then, as you maintain the posture, you allow only roughly 20 percent of the air to escape as you exhale. Then, you inhale only that same relatively small percentage of your lung capacity back in to complete the cycle. Only when you come out of the posture do you return to Normal Breathing.

"Bikram," you are saying, "why are you driving me crazy with these different ways to breathe?" Believe me, my friend, it's for your own good. In some *asanas*, especially the deeper backbends, retaining 80 percent of the breath creates pneumatic pressure inside your lungs. This internal compression helps to stabilize your torso—specifically the whole spinal area—as you bend, so that the body doesn't completely relax. At the same time, you are creating hydraulic pressure in the abdomen (where there are liquids instead of air). With these pneumatic and hydraulic forces, your muscles don't have to sustain the body in these positions entirely on their own. Especially when you are bending backward, unsupported in space, as in Half Moon, this is essential. It will also help you to safely attain and maintain the Floor Bow posture, for example, where you start on the floor, then come upward, against gravity. Even though Camel is a very deep backbend, you're kneeling on the floor and you have your hands on your heels, so it's relatively supported, and we don't need to use the 80/20 technique.

Usually, we'll do each posture two times, one "set," or repetition, right after the other (later in the Sequence we'll rest in *Savasana* between sets). In the Second Set, as I call it, you should try to go a little deeper. The most important thing is to go into these postures as far as you can *while maintaining proper form*. If the form is lost, so is the benefit.

This Sequence should always be performed in front of a full-length mirror. You can wear anything you want, but tighter-fitting clothing is better so you can see clearly in the mirror how and where every part of your body is positioned. Put a towel over your yoga mat for better traction and to absorb the sweat. To maximize the benefits, my Sequence must be done in a hot room—at least 100 degrees. While you may not be able to generate the same powerful, consistent heat we provide in Bikram studios, you can approximate it at home by using a space heater in a small area or running the hot water in the shower and practicing in your bathroom.

Please understand, though, that while I will give you every bit of information and inspiration I can in this book, there's no substitute for going to a Bikram studio and working with one of our certified teachers. Maybe you can come to my Yoga College of India in Los Angeles and we can meet in person! Here you can learn the basics and get an idea of what my Sequence is all about, but to get 100 percent of the benefit, you absolutely need to visit Bikram's Torture Chamber. One of the most important components of my teachings that you can only get in class is:

The Dialogue

Earlier I called my Sequence a song that I wrote to the human body. Well, every song has its lyrics, and the lyrics to my unique song are expressed through the words of the Dialogue. When you attend a Bikram Yoga class, you will notice that the teacher utilizes a distinct set of verbal instructions to guide the class through the 26 postures and two breathing exercises. The directions are the same every time. Twice a year, hundreds of students from all over the world arrive in Los Angeles to attend my Intensive Teacher Training at the International Headquarters of Bikram's Yoga College of India. In nine weeks, they go through nearly 700 rigorous hours of study, practice and application. Only teachers personally certified by me can teach the Sequence, and the most essential requirement, beyond demonstrating an exceptional physical practice and a strong character, is proficiency in relating the Dialogue.

People always say to me—and you may be thinking this right now—"Bikram, don't you know a dialogue is when two people are talking with each other? Since you're the only one talking in class when you give instruction, this should really be called 'the Monologue.'" Let me tell you something: My English may not be perfect, but I know the difference between a monologue and a dialogue. When my teachers and I are talking to a class, telling you what to do, there is a response. From what we can see as you struggle to perform the *asanas* properly, your body is giving us information as well—it is *talking back*. There's a connection, there's communication, and that's why it's a dialogue. You follow me?

Not having the instruction ringing in your ears when you practice with this book is a bit of a loss for you, but to make it up to you, I'll be giving you a bonus in this written format: As we discuss each posture I will give you some specific tips not necessarily contained in the regular Dialogue. From observing thousands of students, I now know exactly where you are likely to go wrong, overcompensate, or just get frustrated and lose your concentration. I'm calling these insights Bikram's Keys, and here's the first one, which applies to every posture.

Bikram's Key

So much of my emphasis is on teaching you how to get into these postures properly, and when you come to me as a beginning student that's what you are concerned with as well. But it's very important to know how to get *out of* the positions, too.

The idea here is to start small and go slow. When you are in a posture and want to make an adjustment to improve your form, make tiny adjustments, not big movements or changes. And come out of the posture very slowly and carefully. If you are new to Bikram Yoga, you are in unexplored territory, and your body is not used to these motions. And even if you have been practicing my Sequence for years, you must remember that when you perform these *asanas*, your body is transforming itself during this 90-minute moving meditation. That's another reason to honor your temple and treat it with care.

Moving deliberately and gracefully also increases your stamina, control, patience and discipline. The effort we make in yoga, the trying—always doing our best despite the pain, the difficulties or obstacles—is an important component; in some ways it *is* yoga. Remember—it's not what you do, it's how you do it. And it's only through that discipline, *trying the right way*, that physical and mental health, peace and Self-Realization can be achieved. Sure, it's hard, but as I said before, the right way is the hard way. So, you see, I don't ask these things of you for no reason.

The Benefits

As we begin to work our way through the Sequence, you'll see that I also describe the most important benefits of the breathing exercise or posture you've just practiced. This leads me to an important and common question: Should you then pick out certain *asanas* and practice them separately to get more of their particular benefit and treat your specific problems or conditions? It's perfectly all right to add extra sets of Awkward Pose, say, to address problems you may be having in your lower spine, but you *must* practice them after you do the entire Sequence. Don't just do them on their own, separate from your regular practice, but instead add them on afterward. That way you'll be fully warmed up, reducing the risk of injury, and you will be getting the full synergistic benefits of the Sequence.

Okay, let's begin.

FIRST BREATHING EXERCISE

Standing Deep Breathing

Pranayama breathing feels strange at first, because your lungs are not used to maximum expansion and contraction. They will feel tight and small, which is perfectly normal. It might even be impossible for you to inhale fully for six full counts (roughly 6 seconds). But with each class, you will find that your breath becomes deeper and fuller. If you have a tiny, Dixie-cup capacity now, soon you will have a big, fat rain barrel.

To begin: Face the mirror with your feet together, pointed straight in front of you, heels together, toes touching. Ridiculously easy as this seems, you might find it hard. Your toes will want to spread themselves out for balance, but don't let them. Keep them together and soon enough you won't feel as if you're about to fall to one side.

Place your hands together and interlace the knuckles. Tuck both hands under your chin, with the knuckles touching the underside of the chin. The elbows are together, and the thumbs are touching the throat. Maintain this contact throughout the exercise.

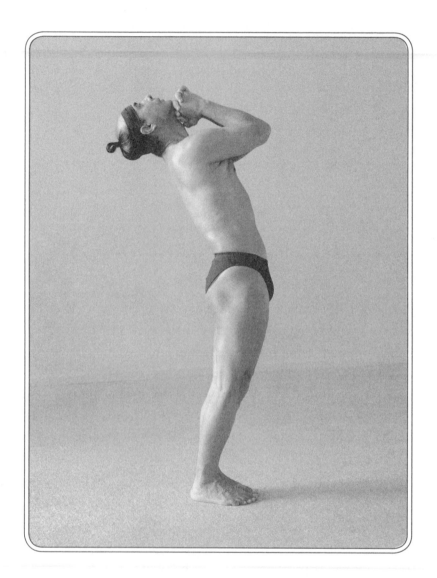

Inhale deeply through the nose, mouth closed, for a slow count of six. Fill up those lungs! At the same time, slowly raise your elbows like seagull wings on either side of your head. Lower your chin downward onto your knuckles, the very center of your two wings. Don't bend forward, just lower your chin. Don't worry if you can't raise your arms above shoulder level at first. Concentrate on pressing the chin against the knuckles. And don't bend your wrists upward to help you get those arms up; keep them straight.

When you've inhaled completely and reached the count of six, drop your head back as far as it can go, keeping your mouth open halfway, while slowly and steadily exhaling for another count of six. As you do that, bring your forearms, elbows and wrists together in front of your face. Keep your chin in firm contact with your knuckles. Force out every last bit of air. Your upturned face and the length of your arms form one straight, even line from the wall behind you to the mirror in front of you.

Do 10 of these inhale-exhale cycles. At the end of the final exhale, bring your head back to an upright position, let your arms fall naturally to your sides and rest a moment. Then raise your arms again to interlock the hands and begin again.

You may feel yourself feeling slightly dizzy as you do this— you're not used to so much oxygen pouring into your system! The dizziness will disappear as you gain more experience. Keep your eyes open the whole time. Otherwise, you might lose your balance and fall over.

Second Set: Rest for a moment, then repeat, doing another series of 10 inhalations and exhalations.

Bikram's Key

The tricky part here is the breathing—you never knew that a mindless, repetitive act could be so complex! Here you must breathe by compressing the throat: As you inhale strongly through your nose, the stream of air should be so powerful that it makes a snoring sound when it hits the back of your throat. Not a pig snort, but a smooth rushing sound. As your throat muscles become more accustomed to this, it will happen naturally. Do the same thing on the exhale, even though the mouth is now open. Force the flow of exiting air upward so that it hits that same snore spot in the back of the throat, underneath the nose, and you'll hear the same rushing sound. In time, the sound you will make while performing this properly will be similar to the sound the air makes when it whispers through a small crack in your car window when you are driving down an open highway.

Benefits

As we've discussed, Standing Deep Breathing teaches you to use up to 100 percent of your lung capacity and in so doing it helps prevent respiratory problems such as bronchitis, emphysema, asthma and shortness of breath. Over time, as the lungs become more elastic and capable of greater expansion, they can actually change the structure of the rib cage that surrounds them, expanding it as well. Like all *pranayama*, Standing Deep Breathing also teaches you to control the breath and to sustain your inhales and exhales rather than gasp. By expanding the lungs, Standing Deep Breathing stimulates circulation, so it wakes up the muscles and the entire body. For that reason, it's a good warm-up before any other kind of exercise.

POSTURE #1:

Half Moon
Ardha-Chandrasana

In Half Moon, you begin to open up the whole skeletal system, including the spine, the neck, the ribs and the scapulae. Your entire body then opens like a beautiful blooming flower. This will include our first backbend, and as soon as we ask students to drop their heads back, a good many of them instantly become afraid. People are terrified to drop their head back; it's as if they think their head is going to fall off onto the floor and roll around behind them. But dropping the head back allows the arms, which will be extended behind you as well, to stretch farther, which is an important part of this posture. Most times, when you reach what seems to be as far as you can go, you can actually go farther, as long as you maintain proper form. It's just your fear that makes you rigid and unable to bend more deeply, especially as a beginner.

If that happens, focus your attention on the base of your neck and tell those muscles to relax. Let go. If you can do that, your head will float back farther than you thought possible just 30 seconds earlier. Look back at the wall behind you; this will also help you to bend more deeply in that direction. Don't worry— your head will in all likelihood remain attached, and in time, you'll overcome that fear.

Flexing the spine this way is incredibly therapeutic, as most of us are constantly bending forward for one reason or another but we rarely, if ever, bend backward. Think about how you are positioned when you are driving your car, working at your computer—

always reaching and leaning forward. In this repetitive, unnatural motion all the nerves emanating from the back of the spine get pushed to one side and the nerves emanating from the front of the spine are constantly compressed—and they hate you for it. This can also lead to imbalances and rigidity, all of which can be eliminated by bending in the opposite direction.

If you have a back problem, then of course you need to take it easy on the backward bending at first. Although it feels dangerous, this motion is actually far less risky than improper forward bending, which we'll cover in the next pose. If you understand how to do it step-by-step, scientifically and intelligently, you won't hurt your back while bending in any direction; you will only help to heal it.

To begin: Stand with your feet together, raise your arms, and bring your hands together, interlocking the fingers in a nice tight grip. Release the index fingers, straightening them and pressing them together—they're going to be the pointed top of the church steeple you'll form with your head and arms. Raise and straighten your arms completely on either side of your head, locking the elbows. Reach upward strongly, pressing the arms against your ears. Keep your head and chin up, looking forward.

Push your hips to the left and, without flexing your arms or legs, slowly bend to your right side as much as possible. Keep your whole body facing front. Keep your arms straight, elbows locked, and don't let your chin sink down into your chest; keep it three inches away. As you stretch your upper body to the right, continue to push both hips directly to the left. Feel the beautiful pull along the left side of your body. (Now you can look in the mirror and see why we call this Half Moon: You're curved, ideally, into a unbroken crescent shape. I've measured my students

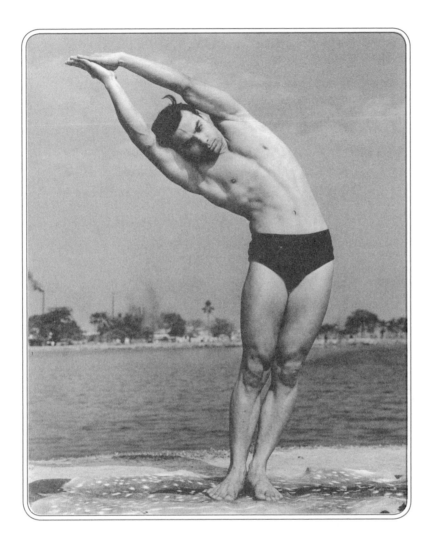

while they are in this posture and the difference in length between the two sides of their torso can be amazing. They can measure 3½ to 4 feet on the stretching side and as little as 8 to 10 inches on the compressed side!)

Stay this way, absolutely still and breathing normally, for 10 full seconds. Then slowly come up to center position, keeping your steeple pointing upward to the sky.

Once again stretch up to the ceiling, then repeat the side-bending motion to your left, pushing your hips out to the right as you move. Keep the arms pressed against the ears, elbows locked. Hold for the 10 count, then come back up to center position.

Note: As in many of these postures, you will almost always do better (bend farther) on one side than the other. Welcome to the human race, my friend; we are all lopsided animals.

Now comes the back bending, and in this part we will be using 80/20 Breathing.

To begin: Stretch up toward the ceiling, lift your torso up out of your hips, inhale 100 percent and hold the breath just for a moment, then slowly drop your head back as far as possible. Easy. Slowly take your arms—still together, still absolutely straight—and upper body backward as much as possible. Begin 80/20 Breathing, inhaling and exhaling only 20 percent of your lung capacity on each breath, keeping 80 percent in your lungs.

Stop bending backward just before you would fall over; your feet should be flat on the floor, weight on your heels. Just as you pushed your hips the opposite way when you bent to the side, now you should push your thighs, stomach and hips forward, countering the backbend and the extension of the arms. Keep the knees and elbows locked. Remain as still as a statue for 10 seconds.

Slowly come back up, keeping your arms and ears together, elbows locked.

Note: We will repeat Half Moon, just not quite yet.

Bikram's Key

The first problem beginners experience in Half Moon's side bends is simultaneously keeping the elbows locked and the chin up. (As I noted before, in the back-bending part, the problem is fear.) The desire and effort may well be there, but the deltoids, scapula and neck have never worked together this way before. At first, keeping all these different parts of your body in alignment is like herding wild monkeys. Plus, in the beginning, it may hurt, too, so beginners are often afraid to do it.

This leads me to one of the most important lessons America has ever taught me: "No pain, no gain." In India, we express the same sentiment as "No money, no honey." Of course it hurts! Contrary to popular belief, pain often means that you are doing something right. Be grateful and be patient. Nobody's telling you to be a martyr or a masochist; I'm just talking about going one small step beyond discomfort. Stretch to the point at which you feel pain, the threshold, and learn from it. Each day that threshold should recede and you'll have to go farther and farther to reach it. Of course, if you have a specific medical problem, you need to regulate yourself accordingly.

Benefits

Half Moon Pose strengthens every muscle in the body's core, especially in the abdomen, and flexes and strengthens the latissimus dorsi, oblique, deltoid and trapezius muscles. It increases the flexibility of the spine comprehensively, from coccyx to neck; promotes proper kidney function; and helps to cure enlargement of the liver and spleen. Half Moon also firms and trims the waistline, hips, abdomen, buttocks and thighs. Give it a couple of weeks and you will probably be able to take that belt in a notch or two. My waist is 28 inches, and I own the same pants I wore 40 years ago—and they still fit. The same can happen for you.

POSTURE #2:

Hands to Feet
Pada-Hasthasana

Since the spine is not quite warmed up yet, you must approach this posture in a slow, controlled manner. (In forward bends such as this one, we use Normal Breathing, not 80/20.) Gravity helps to pull and lengthen your spine. This is also a wonderful stretch for the thigh biceps, what you call hamstrings. Blood rushes to the brain, synovial fluid in your joints begins to flow—this posture wakes up the body and does wonders for the lower back and spine.

To begin: With your feet together nicely, as in Half Moon, lift the torso, then bend forward from the hips, legs straight, stretching and reaching as far down as you can go. When you can no longer keep the legs straight, bend the knees, and reach back and take hold of your heels with your hands, thumbs and forefingers touching the floor. Bend your elbows and press the insides of your forearms completely against the back of your calves. The goal is to eventually touch your elbows together behind your legs.

Stretch your body as much as possible toward the floor. Try to lay your stomach on the tops of your thighs and place the chest on the knees, so that no gaps are visible from the side. Your face is against your legs somewhere below your knees, and your eyes are wide open.

Now slowly push your knees back, keeping your upper and lower bodies glued together and straightening your legs as much

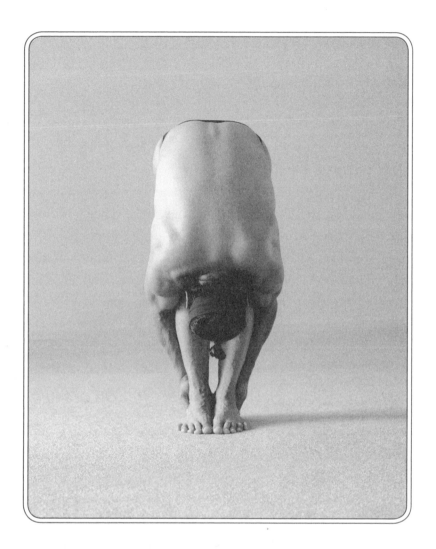

as possible. Your weight should be forward on the toes. Pull on your heels and lift your hips toward the ceiling. Legs straight! Lock the knees! Try harder! I know it hurts behind the knees, but this is a beautiful hurt. This kind of pain is normal, expected and good.

Hold for a 10 count, breathing normally, then let go of the heels and come up slowly and gracefully.

Second Set: Rest for a moment or two, then repeat all three parts of Half Moon (two side stretches and one backbend) and Hands to Feet, holding for 10 seconds on each side, back and front. Then relax.

Bikram's Key

Before you take hold of your heels, bend your knees and place your hands on the floor in front of you. Now, wiggle your hips from side to side a few times. Like yoga *asanas* themselves, this initial warm-up will serve as a diagnostic tool, telling you how tight you are and where. And like performing any and all of the postures, this technique is therapeutic at the same time: It will help to loosen up your ankles, knees and hips, enabling you to deepen your stretch in the posture.

Benefits

Hands to Feet Pose stretches the spine and increases flexibility, as does Half Moon. Both poses firm and trim the lower body, where many problem areas, especially for women, reside. *Pada-Hasthasana* works the muscles, ligaments and tendons of the legs and improves circulation there as well. It also strengthens the glutes, and though this might not be as obvious, it strengthens the upper body and back: the obliques, deltoids and trapezius muscles.

Yoga for Stress

More than 50 years ago my guru, Bishnu Ghosh, said that "mental stress and strain is the cause of all diseases, even infectious ones." Why? Because stress compromises the immune system, your own Department of Defense. Recently, Western medicine has begun to catch up with my guru's wisdom, confirming, among other things, the destructive role of cortisol, a stress hormone, in chronic illness. (Cortisol also contributes to obesity, which I will discuss later.) Diabetes, obesity, hypertension, depression, migraines and chronic pain, just to name a few of the most serious ailments, have all been linked to stress, along with lifestyle habits such as a poor diet.

What is stress? Medical schools will tell you it's "the nonspecific response of the body to any demand, external or internal." Acute stressors are short-term things, like deadlines for taxes, or a big business meeting. Chronic ones include taking care of a terminally ill family member and having a high-pressure job. With either kind of stress, the body is sent into emergency overdrive, the "fight-or-flight response," and our bodies release chemicals such as adrenaline and cortisol to help us cope or respond to the stressor. An adrenaline rush, for example, can help us run away faster from danger. (The fight-or-flight response also raises the heart and breathing rates, and directs blood away from normal functions such as digestion so it can be used for emergency responses.)

Over time and with repeated emergencies—or at least events and conditions that we *perceive* as stressful—the body becomes overwhelmed by the constant release of these hormones and their acidic, corrosive effects. We're exhausted, and the immune system, endocrine system and nervous system cannot function at their best, which causes high blood pressure, sleep disorders, chronic headaches, neck tension, backaches, depression and anxiety.

With the natural science of yoga we tap into the body's intrinsic healing system, calming and reintegrating the mind, body and emotions. Through the postures and the breath work in Hatha Yoga, we take back control and turn off the fight-or-flight response and its flood of bad biochemistry. Here's just a little of the recent clinical confirmation of this by Western scientists, proof of how well Hatha Yoga returns the body to equilibrium.

In 2005, a German study compared groups of women who were acutely distressed over a three-month period. Those who practiced yoga showed significantly lower levels of cortisol compared to those in the control group, and made significant decreases in their levels of perceived stress, anxiety, fatigue and depression. They reported higher levels of well-being and they improved physically as well; women suffering from headaches or back pain experienced marked relief. Countless other studies have shown yoga's effectiveness in stress management. You don't need an anti-anxiety drug with potentially gruesome side effects. Instead, get up off that couch and heal yourself by practicing Hatha Yoga.

POSTURE #3:

Awkward Pose
Utkatasana

Awkward Pose is a powerful strengthening posture, and when done with Deep Breathing, Half Moon and Hands to Feet, it also concludes a sort of warm-up section in which you generate internal heat and loosen the muscles.

Sometimes people who come to my classes are expecting Sun Salutations, which other teachers may use as a warm-up early in their sequences. The first few postures and *pranayama* allow me to dispense with them. Can you think of another reason we don't need Sun Salutes? *The heat!* In the studio or at home (after you turn it into a sweatshop), you will be plenty warm, believe me.

Awkward Pose is very challenging for a lot of people, so it's good for instilling discipline and integrating control of the mind with the actions of the body. Your mind may start yelling at you, "Get out, get out, get out!" But meanwhile, of course, I'm yelling at you, "Chest up! Sit down! Stay there!" And who are you going to listen to? That's right—me.

To begin: Stand with your feet about 6 inches apart, or the space of both fists together on the floor between your feet. Raise your arms straight out in front of you, parallel with the floor, palms down and fingers together. There should be 6 inches between your two arms, and the wrists should also be 6 inches apart. Don't let the arm muscles go slack; keep them nice and tight.

Now, keeping your heels flat on the floor, exhale completely and sit down as deeply as you can, as if you are sitting in an imag-

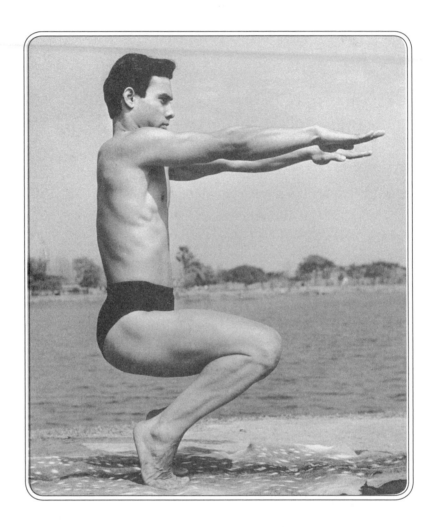

inary chair behind you, until your thighs are parallel to the floor. (If you can't sit down deeply enough to bring your thighs parallel at first, don't be concerned. Only the very limber among you will be able to do this straight off.)

Keeping your weight in your heels, lift your chest up and lean your upper body backward while stretching your fingertips toward the mirror in front of you. The compression of the spine in this posture is similar to that in Cobra Pose, which we'll get to later. Keep 6 inches of space between the toes, heels, knees and hands. Count to 10 slowly.

Come up slowly, with your arms in the same position, and keep going, raising all the way up onto your toes, and locking your knees by squeezing the thigh muscles. Now bend your knees and—still up on your tippy toes—sit down again, spine straight, back flat, stomach sucked in, until your thighs are parallel to the floor. Imagine you have a wall behind you and you are pressing your back against it. You'll be straight when you feel as if you are tipping backward slightly. Your heels are as high off the ground as you can make them. Stay in the position for 10 seconds. This is a killer, but stick with it even as your leg muscles are trembling. Please remember to breathe.

Slowly come back to standing flat. Your arms are still stretching forward, toward the mirror.

Now we come to the third phase: This time, just rise up on your toes a little bit, then squeeze the knees and thighs tightly together, suck in your stomach, and sink slowly down, all the way, until you are sitting on your heels. Your back is straight, sliding against the same imaginary wall as in the second part. Your arms are parallel with the floor. Stay here for 10 seconds, then come back up, back flat, stomach in, and slowly lower the arms and feet together. *Ahhhhh . . .*

Second Set: Rest for a moment, then repeat the pose, holding all three parts for at least 10 seconds each.

Bikram's Key

In the first two phases of this posture, your knees will try to move closer to each other. Don't let them—remember to keep

them 6 inches apart. The hands also have a way of floating upward as you sink downward, so keep them in check as well. To do
this properly, your arms must be parallel with the floor. Keep
them tight, elbows locked, five fingers together. Another key:
Keep the stomach sucked in and tight.

Benefits

Awkward Pose will tone and shape your legs like nobody's
business. And quickly: The definition and strength you gain here
are among yoga's fastest results. This posture is such a great warm-
up in part because it stimulates circulation, sending blood roar-
ing to your lower extremities. If you suffer from chronically cold
feet, that will be over. It also helps relieve rheumatism and arthritis in the legs, and helps to cure slipped discs and other problems in the lower spine. Awkward Pose also promotes laser-beam
concentration.

POSTURE #4:

Eagle Pose
Garurasana

In the first three postures we've stretched the spine and strengthened the body in many ways. Now we move into a compression posture—you are going to squeeze your body like you've never squeezed anything before. Stopping the compression will release all the tension that's built up in the previous poses and open up all the major joints in the body: hips, knees, ankles, shoulders, elbows and wrists.

To begin: Standing with your feet together, extend your arms overhead, then swing them back down and cross them at the elbows, using the gentle momentum to help you bring the right arm under the left and wrap the right arm as far around the other one as you can. Twist the arms together like ropes, forearms intertwined in front of you with no daylight between them. Now place the palms flat against each other, thumbs toward your face and finger pads pressing against the pads on the opposite hand. Keeping your head up, still facing forward, try to pull your elbows down to your chest so your fingertips go below your nose. That's the beak of the Eagle.

Now, find a point in the mirror in front of you and concentrate on it, keeping all of your attention there. Bend your knees and sit down, lowering yourself about six inches toward an imaginary chair behind you. Shift all your weight to your left leg.

Now slowly lift up your right leg straight in front of you, then reach it over the left thigh and wrap the right calf and foot

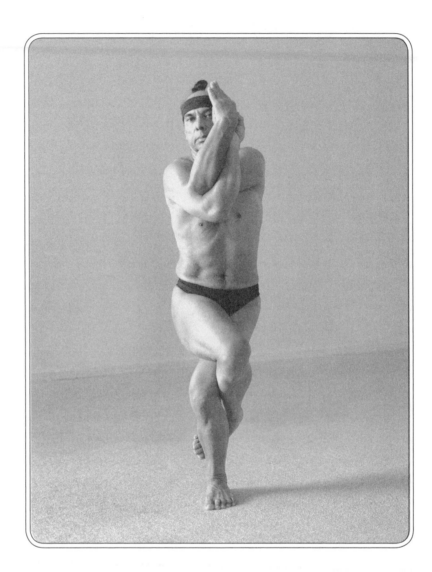

around the calf of the standing leg, your left. Just like with the arms, you want the calves wrapped around each other, tight like ropes.

Sink down deeper on the standing leg, as far as possible. Lean your upper body back and squeeze your knees, ankles and thighs as if you were cracking walnuts between them all. All the time you are breathing and pulling down with the arms and concentrating on your spot in the mirror. Stay still for 10 seconds.

Come up, untangle all your arms and legs, then do the posture in reverse, left arm under right, left leg up and around the right, for another 10 seconds.

Second Set: Rest a moment, then repeat the posture, holding it for 10 seconds on each side.

Bikram's Key

You might not be able to wrap your arms properly at first, but that's okay. This is a strange and difficult position and, especially if you're a man, with bigger shoulders, forearms and biceps, the full braiding will be difficult. In any case, your work is the same: Pulling down continuously with the arms will develop the flexibility you need in the shoulders and slowly stretch out all those tight places in your neck and shoulders, where so many of us hold our tension.

To help you wrap your legs tighter, try this technique, the counterpart to the one we used to get the arms braided together by first swinging them overhead. After you bend the legs, lift your right one up really high and reach *as far left* with it as you can before you bring it back down and wrap it around the left calf. Also: Try to simultaneously lean back and sit down deeper, lowering your center of gravity and keeping more of your weight in your heel.

Benefits

Eagle is the only posture that opens up the 14 largest joints in the skeletal system (seven on each side of the body) in such a short time—just 10 seconds! Beyond improving flexibility in the hips, knees, ankles and the rest, Eagle also supplies fresh blood to the reproductive system and sex organs, plus the kidneys, which increases sexual vitality and helps clear up reproductive problems. It tones the calves, thighs and hips, while in the upper body it strengthens the latissimus dorsi, trapezius, and deltoid muscles.

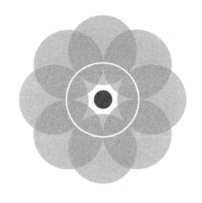

CHAPTER SEVEN

Postures 5-12

*Plus: Yoga for Insomnia,
and Yoga for Obesity
and Weight Control*

POSTURE #5:

Standing Head to Knee
Dandayamana-Janushirasana

At this point we go into the three postures that comprise the standing, one-legged concentration series. This is where you begin to employ one of the most misunderstood principles in Bikram Yoga. It's also an apt metaphor for living the life of a yogi, with determination and balance. Here's how I express this principle in my Dialogue: *"Lock the knee! Lock the knee! Lock the knee!"*

Remember how I told you earlier that one of your biggest problems in America is *"no problem,"* that many of you don't really have many serious challenges to deal with in your lives? Well, now you have a problem: You will not be able to lock your knee. It sounds so simple, but to continuously contract the thigh muscles, lock your standing knee and balance evenly on a solid, unwavering leg for even 10 seconds is nearly impossible for most beginning students. But unless you can do this, you can't really do Bikram Yoga. Here's why: If the thigh muscles remain slack, you will create unnecessary compression in the knee joint, eventually causing damage. When you engage the quadriceps femoris muscles, the tendons and ligaments of the knee become active and pull bone away from bone, strengthening and rehabilitating the joint. This is a strong example of why concentration is so important to practicing Hatha Yoga and successfully healing the body.

What's more, if you cannot lock the knee, you won't ever find Self-Realization. People say I am a hard-ass teacher, and it's true. But in this yoga class and in life, you have to experience hell on

Earth so that you may eventually reach heaven. Struggle instills discipline, so we can begin to control our minds. Suffering breeds compassion. It sounds simplistic, but until you've actually stood on your own leg with your knee safely and powerfully locked like a solid piece of concrete, truly believing that you don't even *have* a knee, you won't be able to find inner peace, love and happiness. This is why I always have to scream at my students to push them toward this goal. I tell my students, "When you die, I will jump up and down on your grave, shouting 'Lock the damn knee!'"

To begin: Stand upright with your feet together. Shift your weight to your left foot and lock the left knee. The thigh muscles are contracted and hard; the whole leg is one solid piece, like a lamppost. I'll say it again: Locking the standing knee at all times during the posture is essential—if the standing knee bends, you get no benefits and risk potential injury.

Now lift your right knee up high, bend forward, reach out with both hands, and interlace your fingers underneath the ball of your right foot, about three inches below the tips of your toes. Hold on tight. (You may want to wipe your hands on the towel before you attempt this so the foot doesn't slip out of your grasp.)

Now raise the extended leg so that it's exactly parallel to the floor, and lock that knee. Flex your foot so the toes are facing you. As you do this, you are also pushing the heel forward, away from you. Both legs are hard and tight.

This is hard. It may take you some time to be able to do it properly, without cheating. Only when you can achieve this— getting your two legs locked with them forming a 90-degree angle—may you progress to the next part of the posture: Bend your elbows and pull the ball of your foot and the toes toward you with all your power. The elbows are pointing down to the floor,

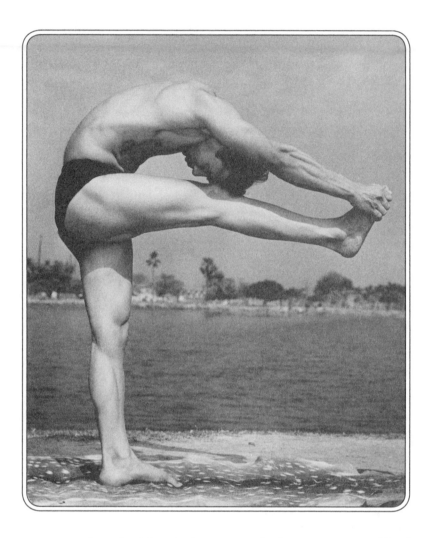

not out to the sides like chicken wings. Before you attempt Head to Knee, the elbows must first go below the calf muscle. Now pull hard as you kick the heel away. Both legs are completely straight, both knees locked. Now bend your torso forward, tuck your chin into your chest, and try to touch your forehead to the knee. Fix your concentration on a spot on the floor to help you keep your balance initially, until you can keep your eyes on your belly button without taking yourself out of the posture. Keep your stomach sucked in, creating a compression of the abdominal wall. Stay here for 60 seconds.

Slowly straighten up and come out of the posture in exactly the same way you came into it, only in reverse. Then begin on the other side by locking the right leg, bending forward, and picking up the left foot, then extending and locking that leg as well. Hold the pose for another 60 seconds.

Second Set: Rest for a moment, then repeat the posture, holding for 60 seconds on each side.

Bikram's Key

When you fall out of this posture at any point—and you will—you must start all over again, at the very first part. Why? As with all the postures, learning Standing Head to Knee is a process. That's what's important, not the outcome. Remember: The posture is never the object when practicing yoga—the body is the object. We move forward step-by-step, building the complete and correct form slowly and sequentially, brick by brick. This posture is a diagnostic tool that shows your levels of focus and determination, both to your teacher and to you. Just as Half Moon tells me immediately how strong, flexible and balanced you are, standing head to knee instantly reveals how much concentration power you have developed. Feed your own Bengal tiger and your own inner bulldog!

Benefits

When you learn to lock the knee properly, this posture improves the flexibility of the sciatic nerves and strengthens the hamstrings and leg muscles. Plus it works the muscles of the back, the biceps and the triceps. When you touch your forehead to your knee, you create front-side compression, so you are also squeezing and flushing out the internal abdominal organs, such as the gall bladder, pancreas and spleen, as well as the uterus and ovaries.

POSTURE #6:

Standing Bow Pose
Dandayamana-Dhanurasana

As we move to the second stop in this one-legged series, a word about balance. In other yoga methods the instructors sometimes recommend that you use a wall, a chair or another prop to keep you from falling over while you're in the early stages of balance training. But I say you don't need these props, even if you're a beginner. You'll actually progress faster if you stick it out on your own, and when you rely on props, even though it *seems* like you're progressing, you're not really learning the posture. Take away that wall or chair and you can't do it. You're building with fake bricks. Remember: Proper form is essential and depth is relative, especially as a beginner. The only way is the right way and the right way is the hard way.

To begin: Stand on your left leg, knee locked. Bend your right leg at the knee and reach behind you with your right hand, palm turned up facing the ceiling. Grab the foot from the inside around the ankle, cupping the instep in your hand, fingertips on the top of your foot. Don't worry; everyone messes this up at first.

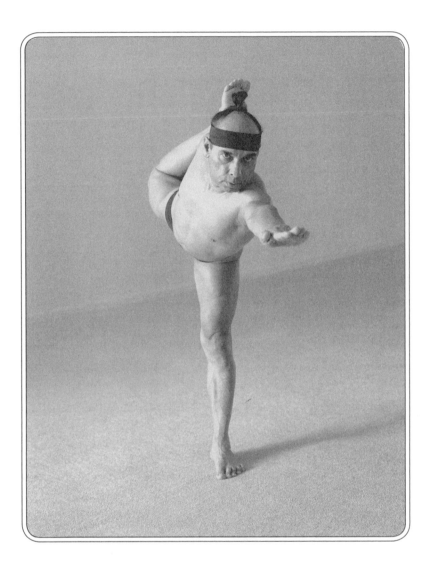

The sole of the foot is facing up. Your right kneecap is facing the floor.

Raise your left arm up straight out in front of you, fingers together and pointing toward the ceiling. Bring your knees together, and stretch up as far as possible to try and touch your shoulder to your chin without moving your head. Keeping your whole torso and extended left arm in one solid piece, roll forward from the hips to the fingertips, until your abdomen is parallel to the floor.

As you do this, you're stretching *forward* with the arm and kicking the right foot *back* with all your strength. Push it back smoothly, don't jerk it, and push the foot out powerfully against your cupped hand. (Keep the right arm and shoulder relaxed.) Arch your head and spine backward as you pivot your torso forward. Your body is bending just like a bow when it's being drawn by an archer. Creating this tension is what keeps you balanced in the posture. It's Newton's Third Law of Motion. For every action, there is an equal and opposite reaction. If you feel yourself starting to fall out of the pose, kick back even more while stretching your arm forward more as well (and maintaining your breathing). These actions seem counterintuitive, but increased, equal pressure in those two places makes your bow more taut, which will restore your balance. Don't think about balance—just concentrate on kicking back harder and the balance will take care of itself.

Kick higher. It may hurt a little in the back of your standing leg, but don't be afraid—keep that knee locked. Eventually you will achieve a perfect standing split. Look in the mirror and make sure your lifted knee isn't sticking out to the side; it should be invisible behind your body. Your lifted arm stays right alongside your head at all times. Stay poised there, beautiful and graceful, for 60 seconds. If you fall out of the posture, you'll have plenty of time to attempt it again.

Now do the pose on the other side.

Second Set: Rest for a moment, then repeat the posture, holding for 60 seconds on each side.

Bikram's Key

Don't dive forward into this position too fast. Everyone wants to look beautiful in the finished pose, so they rush to get into it. Take the time to get yourself firmly grounded and set on your standing leg before you bring your body forward and down. When you do begin to move, take your time and stay in control. Let the power of the kick do the work. If you are unable to bring your chest, abdomen and stomach down parallel to the floor, allow yourself to fall gently forward out of the posture. Don't worry; your extended arm will stop you from hitting the floor if you momentarily lose control.

Benefits

Only the Standing Bow moves all the blood from one side of the body to the other, then back again. It uses the compression and extension, and then the release, that I described earlier—the Hoover Dam effect—systematically bringing fresh blood and oxygen to all the organs and glands. It develops balance, increases the size and elasticity of the rib cage, firms the abdominal wall and upper thighs, tightens upper arms, hips and buttocks and improves the flexibility and strength of the lower spine. Mentally, Standing Bow builds patience, determination and concentration.

POSTURE #7:

Balancing Stick
Tuladandasana

As in full inversions, including Headstand or Handstand, in this posture you lower your heart below your hips, which sends large amounts of blood rushing into the heart. It's like giving yourself an intentional heart attack, so you become stronger and never have one of the accidental and unwelcome kind. And despite what you may think, this is actually more demanding than those other inversions; it can be much easier to stay in a Headstand for an hour than it is to do this one-legged Balancing Stick correctly for 10 seconds.

To begin: Stand with your feet together. Stretch your arms up over your head and interlock the fingers, index fingers pointing up to form your steeple. The arms are right behind your ears. Stretch your upper body backward, so that the chest puffs up and forward. Now take a big step to the front with your right leg. Come up on the toes of your back foot. Look forward into the mirror.

Now, with your body one solid piece from the fingers to your toes, knees and elbows locked, pivot directly forward on your hip joint while simultaneously raising your left leg behind you, toes pointed. Again, your abdomen should be exactly parallel to the floor as are your outstretched arms and extended back leg: one straight line. Both knees are locked. You know what that means, don't you? *Locked.* Solid, concrete, one piece, like a lampost— you have no knee.

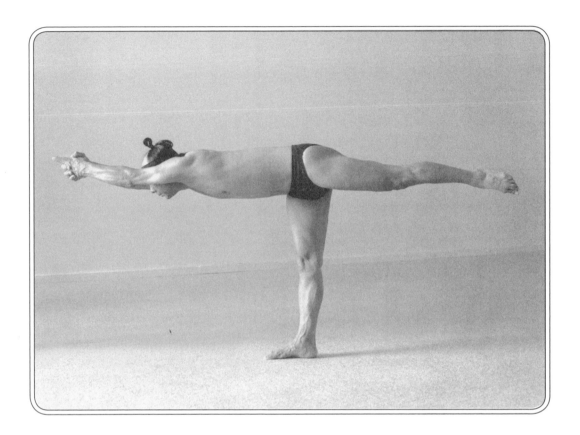

You may not be able to come all the way forward today and form that perfect T-shape. That's okay; just go as far as you can, and stay there for a full 10 seconds.

Then step back to center. Feel like a nice rest after all that work? Not yet, honey. Keep the arms outstretched over your head, biceps behind the ears, fingers interlocked. Now instead of relaxing, do the pose on the other side, and hold it for 10 seconds.

Return to center; lower the arms. *Now* rest.

Second Set: Repeat the posture on each side, then rest again. You've earned it, my friend.

Bikram's Key

This posture is all about locking the body into one solid line. To do that, imagine a tug of war: Someone is pulling your back foot toward the wall with all his might and someone else is pulling your outstretched hands as hard as she can in the opposite direction, toward the mirror in front of you. Again, this puts you into natural human traction, stretching the spine from coccyx to neck.

Benefits

The forward tilt of your torso sends high-speed blood pouring into the heart, especially the neglected lower region, cleaning out the veins and all the arteries, strengthening the heart muscle. The same rejuvenating flood rushes into the brain as well. It is also one of the best exercises for bad posture. And by perfecting body control and balance it strengthens your powers of concentration.

Yoga for Insomnia

Maybe it's indigestion, something you ate that now torments your stomach and keeps you tossing and turning. Maybe it's overstimulation from drinking caffeine during the day, or just the garden-variety stress of 21st-century life— mental indigestion—that's got you up at night. All of these reasons add up to more than 35 million prescriptions a year in the United States for sleep medications.

Throw away those pills with their risk of dependency and bizarre side effects. Did you know that some people actually get up in their drugged sleep and eat like pigs or even drive their cars while they're on these medicines? Now *that's* a nightmare.

Yoga is the natural, effective prescription for insomnia. I once helped a woman named Mrs. Murphy, who hadn't slept well for *18 years*. Prescription medications didn't work. Her husband told me, "She's tired all the time, she's cranky all the time; you must help us!"

So, long story short, I taught her yoga for just one month, and now her husband has another complaint: "Mr. Choudhury, what are you doing to my wife? She's sleeping all the time, fourteen hours a night!"

"Relax, my friend," I told him. "She's just catching up; she has to recharge her batteries after eighteen years. Let her make up some, and soon she will be fine and you'll have your beautiful wife back. Then she's going to wear you out!" And that's what happened.

How does yoga prevent insomnia?

✦   As we've discussed elsewhere, yoga calms the sympathetic ner- vous system, which generates adrenaline (and the fight-or-flight response). With less of this hormone coursing through your veins, you can take your rest in peace. Since yoga *asanas* were originally designed to calm the body and quiet the mind, this makes complete sense.

✦ Yoga stimulates circulation, including sending more blood to the sleep center of the brain.

✦ *Pranayama,* or breathing exercises, also have a calming effect on the brain, reducing anxiety and arousal, and thus promoting sleep. In a study at the Harvard Medical School by Sat Bir Khalsa, PhD, insomniacs practiced daily meditative *pranayama* at home for eight weeks. After that, *all* of the subjects reported improvements in how long it took them to fall asleep, how often they woke up during the night, and their ability to get back to sleep.

✦ You may actually need less sleep when you practice yoga due to the elimination of toxins from the body, which gives you more high-octane gas for your engine. Your mileage may vary, but it will definitely be improved. Take me: I barely sleep at all and I have more energy than anyone in the world! Ask anyone who knows me; it's true.

Rabbit Pose (posture #22; see page 195) is especially good for insomnia; however, your overall, comprehensive practice is the best cure for any and all sleep disorders. Besides all the scientific reasons I cite above, giving your best effort in my heated Torture Chamber will definitely kick your butt! After that, you will definitely sleep. Sweet dreams, my friend.

POSTURE #8:

Standing Separate Leg Stretching Pose

Dandayamana-Bibhaktapada-Paschimotthanasana

In this posture you will use your strength to create flexibility. Notice how the power you generate by pulling on your heels stretches the legs, hips and spine. Remember to tighten the thigh muscles—they should be hard like rocks!—to help lock the knees.

To begin: Start with your feet together. Raise your arms overhead, palms together, and take a b-i-g step to the right, at least 4 feet. Let me give you some incentive to really spread your legs: The wider the stance, the easier this stretch will become. As you step, lower your arms out to the sides, parallel to the floor. Turn in both feet so they are slightly pigeon-toed.

Bend forward, then reach down to grab your feet from the outside, underneath your heels, thumbs on the outside. All five fingers are together. Pulling hard on the heels, come forward from the lower spine and touch your forehead to the floor, as close to the body as possible. Your weight is on your toes; very little is on the forehead. Your back isn't rounded, it's perfectly straight. Stay like this for at least 20 seconds, eyes open.

Okay, that's the ideal. For you, maybe, we're in fantasyland. But this isn't as hard as you think. Your weight and the way you position your body will do most of the work, if you let them. If

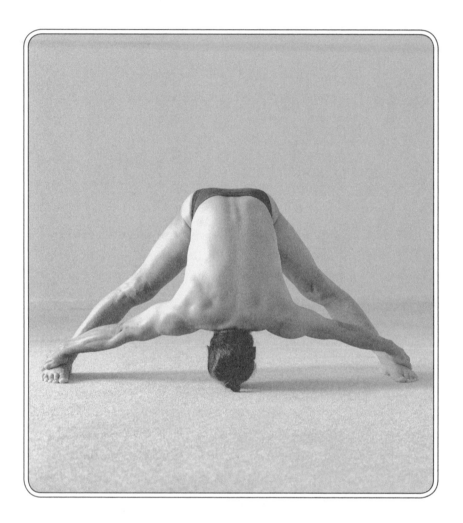

you find this difficult, reach down and put your hands on the floor in front of you, about 12 inches apart (instead of taking hold of your heels). Legs are still straight, knees locked. Now bend the elbows up toward the ceiling and roll your body forward like a wheel, reaching for the floor with your forehead. Still a ways away? Lucky for you there are extra, untapped inches in all your tight muscles and tendons. With repeated stretching you will soon feel yourself unwinding like a winch on a crane, lowering your wrecking ball head smoothly to the floor.

If, on the other hand, you can touch your forehead to the floor easily, take a shorter step to the side at the beginning; this will make the stretch more challenging. In either case, hold for at least 20 seconds.

Now slowly straighten up, then step your feet back together.

Second Set: Rest, then repeat the pose, holding for another 20 seconds, minimum.

Bikram's Key

If you're having trouble grabbing underneath your heels, try grabbing anywhere underneath the outside edge of your foot, even if it's just with your fingertips. And keep your weight forward on the toes.

Benefits

A while back we talked about sciatica, a very common back problem. This posture is like kryptonite for sciatica! That's because it stretches and strengthens those poor crushed and shriveled sciatic nerves, as well as all the tendons in the legs. Standing Separate Leg Stretching also massages the internal abdominal organs and the small and large intestines, and gives you added flexibility in the pelvis, ankles, hip joints and especially in the last five vertebrae of the spine.

POSTURE #9:

Triangle Pose
Trikanasana

The first thing you'll notice, I'll bet, about this posture is that it's not the Triangle you're used to seeing. Most teachers of non–Bikram Yoga here in the United States do a straight-legged version, while in mine, the forward leg is bent. I have no quarrel with the other method—really!—it's an apples and oranges situation, as you say here. With the legs straight, Triangle is more of a stretching pose. But at this point in my Sequence, you don't need that so much. The way I teach it, Triangle is more of an integrative pose, in that you have to use a tremendous amount of balance and strength as well as flexibility—and the breathing, of course—to maintain the posture. Challenging on a physical level, it's also extremely demanding in the way your mind must micromanage your body in so many ways simultaneously. Your body has got to constantly adjust and respond. Once again, the right way is the hard way.

Whether this makes it an apple or an orange, I leave to you. Either way, Triangle addresses every system, organ and gland of the body. A to Z, 360 degrees. As a result, it may be the most therapeutic *asana* of all (see "Benefits").

To begin: Take a wide stance, at least 4 feet, like we did in the last posture, and extend your arms straight out to the sides, palms down. Pivot on your right foot, turning it 90 degrees out to the side. Now bend the right knee until the back of your right

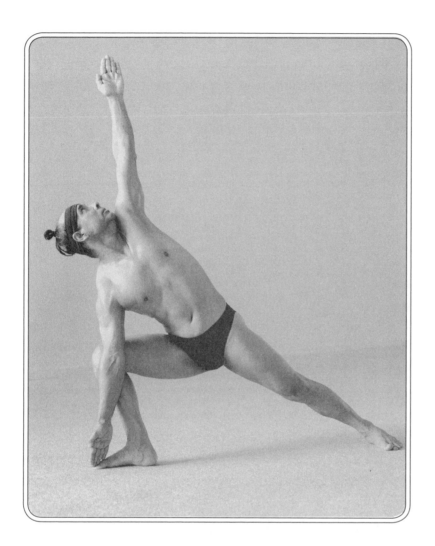

thigh is parallel to the floor. Your spine stays straight and your face, body and hips are still facing front.

Move both arms at the same time, keeping the torso stable and spine straight. Turn the palms forward and reach down with the right arm, while equally and simultaneously reaching up with the left, placing the elbow in front of the right knee and touching the tips of your fingertips to the floor between the big toe and the second toe of your right foot. There shouldn't be any weight or pressure on the fingers; you're just barely touching the floor. Your weight should be on your bent leg. Push gently backward on the knee with the elbow to open up the right hip.

Turn your head and look up. Move your chin to touch your left shoulder so that the profile of your face becomes visible in the mirror in front of you. Your left arm, still straight and still in line with the right one, is now pointing up at the sky (okay, the ceiling). Reach even higher with the left arm and fingers. Stay here for 20 seconds. Breathe! This posture helps create a marriage between the heart and lungs—and breathing deeply and consistently ensures that it's a happy one.

Now move your arms back to parallel as you straighten the bent leg and come back to your wide stance. Turn the right foot back in so it's facing straight ahead once more. Keep those arms up, of course.

Now turn your left foot out and create the Triangle on the other side. Again, one side is always going to be easier. This posture is a killer for beginners, especially those with tight hips, but it doesn't take long to develop the necessary strength and depth.

Second Set: Repeat the posture, first the right leg, then the left leg.

Bikram's Key

If you put weight on the fingertips touching the floor, the posture and benefits are ruined. So don't put any pressure on them! Just touch them there lightly.

Benefits

What doesn't Triangle do? It improves every single bone, muscle, joint, tendon and internal organ, and it revitalizes nerves, veins and tissues. No other pose increases strength and flexibility in the hips as well as this one, and you can easily feel how it tones the muscles on the sides of your torso, including the obliques and the intercostals. Flexing and strengthening the last five vertebrae in this posture can alleviate crooked spines, as well as rheumatism and lower back pain. Triangle also benefits the heart and lungs, forcing them to work together like an arranged marriage in India. They may not want to be together at first, but they have to be. No choice.

POSTURE #10:

Standing Separate Leg Head to Knee Pose

Dandayamana-Bibhaktapada-Janushirasana

As in many other postures, the goal here—bringing your head to your knee with the legs straight—can be difficult if not impossible to achieve at first. One thing to remember in all these situations is that breathing deeply will help you get further into any stretch. So inhale and exhale fully, keeping the breath under your control, and with each exhale, try to go a little deeper into the pose.

To begin: Start with your feet together, arms overhead. Palms together, thumbs crossed, elbows locked. Take a big step sideways to the right; at least three feet. As in the Standing Separate Leg Stretching, taking a wider stance here will make this stretch easier to accomplish. Turn the right foot out to the right side, same as in Triangle, but this time also turn your hips and torso to face the right. Your left foot is at a 45-degree angle.

Keeping both legs absolutely straight, stretch up toward the ceiling, then curl your body up and out, over and down, bringing the forehead to the right knee. You revolve downward like a wheel on an axle. Look at your belly button and exhale 100 percent of the air in your lungs. Suck in the stomach to create compression and stabilize the spine. Your clasped hands should rest gently on the floor in front of your foot, with the arms and elbows straight. Square your hips so they become parallel to the floor.

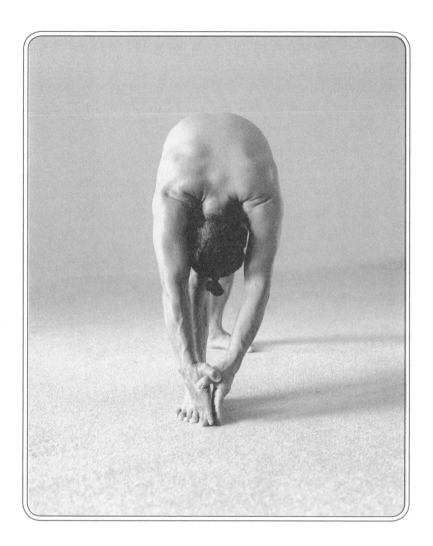

If you cannot do this for the first few weeks or so, simply bend the right knee as far as you need to in order to get the forehead to touch. But the forehead shouldn't go lower than the knee. Now, to achieve the ideal posture, you can spread your fingertips on the floor in front of your toes and push into the floor, elbows locked, and push on that knee with your forehead, straightening the bent leg, eventually, into the locked-knee position. You'll feel the stretch in the back of the knee. Count to 10 as you breathe, eyes open.

Straighten up in the exact reverse of how you went into the pose, and turn back to the center. Maintain your wide-legged stance. Now pivot on the heels, turning the left foot out this time, and reverse the pose.

Second Set: Rest a moment, then repeat the posture, holding for 10 seconds on each side.

Bikram's Key

You're an educated person; I know you know what your forehead is. But an amazing number of people tell me they can't touch their forehead to their knees, then when I look, they are reaching with their nose or their chin, not their forehead. Strange. However, touching the forehead to the knees is simple: Tuck in the chin and keep it there as you move toward the knee; that will keep you from sticking your nose or chin where it doesn't belong. Eyes on the belly button. Many benefits are lost if the forehead and knee come apart, so remember to bend your knee as much as you need to so that they touch.

Benefits

Standing Separate Leg Head to Knee Pose trims the abdomen, waistline, hips, buttocks and thighs. It massages and compresses the thyroid gland, which helps to regulate the metabolism and the immune system.

POSTURE #11:

Tree Pose
Tadasana

One of my favorite all-time students is a woman named Emmy. She's been a teacher for me for 35 years now. But when she first started studying with me, she had done yoga in other places and she used to argue with me about how I was teaching some of the postures, including this one. In many other American schools you'll see students tucking the raised foot into the inner thigh in Tree, not resting it on the front of the thigh as I teach it. "I didn't learn to do it that way," Emmy would say. "Why are you making us to do it this way?"

And of course, I would sweetly tell her, "Shut up, and do what I tell you."

Emmy decided to do a little tour of India, where she studied with a whole bunch of teachers, including Mr. Iyengar. And she wrote me a postcard from India and told me: "You're right; everywhere I go here, even in the hospitals where they are using yoga as therapy, they do the postures just the way you taught us. It turns out the best yoga in the world is in Beverly Hills!" No kidding, honey.

The way I'm going to teach this pose to you, it's more of a hip opener. At the same time, it doesn't put a lot of pressure on the knee, so it's safe. This balancing action also prepares you for Toe Stand, the very powerful posture we will do next. If we were doing the traditional 84 postures, these two in combination would

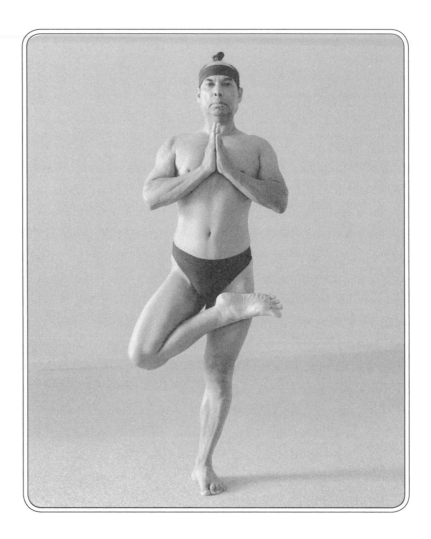

prepare the body to do the Lotus pose. But most Westerners have very tight hips, which in turn puts unnecessary strain on the knees in Lotus. So I don't use it in the Sequence.

To begin: Standing with your feet together, find a spot to focus on in front of you, then lift your right foot and balance on the left leg. Reach down with both hands and grab the right foot.

Slowly, so as not to ruin your balance, raise the foot and bring it to rest as high as you can on the front of your left thigh or hip. The outside of the right foot is the part making contact with the upper leg, not the sole. As the flexibility in your hips increases, you will be able to take the foot all the way up to groin level and leave it there.

Stand up straight and lock the standing knee. Now push both hips forward, and try to move the right knee downward and back toward the wall behind you. Ideally, it will be directly in line with the other knee, though that may not happen for some time. Straighten your back and bring your hands together in the center of your chest, in prayer position. If your foot won't stay on your thigh and keeps falling off, you can reach down with your left hand and just hold it in place, palm facing forward. Leave your right hand in the center of your chest, as if you were praying with one hand. Stay here, as still as possible, for 60 seconds (or longer, if you can).

Lower the right foot and return to standing. Shake out the leg that was bent and raised, then straighten it and lock the knee. Raise the left foot, repeating the posture on the other side.

Note: We do not do a Second Set of Tree, but move right into Toe Stand, which we'll also do for one set (practicing the posture just once on each leg).

Bikram's Key

Many of you keep the raised foot in place by cheating: You stick your butt backward like a duck, which helps keep the foot from falling off its perch. The way to combat this cheating is by slowly turning your head sideways to glance in the mirror. Once you see how undignified you look with your buttocks protruding this way, you will want to perform the posture correctly.

Benefits

The Tree Pose improves posture and balance and increases the flexibility of the ankles and knees as well as the hip joints. By strengthening the internal oblique muscles, it prevents hernia.

POSTURE #12:

Toe Stand
Padangustasana

The knees are the weakest link in the human body and one of the most difficult parts to strengthen. By doing this powerful posture you not only strengthen them, but also develop the yogi's discipline, determination and patience. Toe Stand looks intimidating, but you are now sufficiently warmed up and focused to do it, and I promise you, your knees will not break. (*Note:* If you have a very recent injury or an acute knee problem, just do a Second Set of Tree instead.)

To begin: Stand with your feet together, and focus your attention on a spot on the floor 4 feet in front of you. Like in Tree Pose, shift your weight onto the right leg and lift your left foot up onto your right thigh. Bring your hands to prayer position in the middle of your chest. (Whether or not you actually choose to pray is your own business, and nobody else's.)

Now bend the right knee and lower yourself on one leg as far as you can go with your hands still together. Bend forward from the lower spine, reaching down and placing the fingertips of both hands on the floor for support. Then continue to sink down slowly until your coccyx bone is sitting on your right heel. Your right foot isn't flat on the ground; you're balancing yourself on the ball of the foot. Keep your chin down and your eyes on the floor in front of you.

Now straighten the spine, and suck in your stomach. Pick up the right hand and put it back in prayer position on your chest.

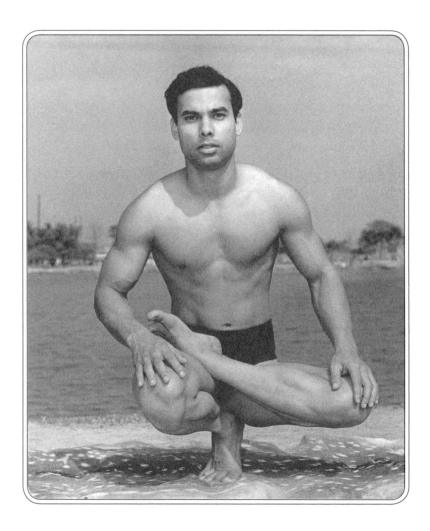

Stabilize yourself again and then move the other hand to meet the first. Slowly look up, then raise your chin to parallel. Stay here for 10 seconds. (Start counting after you achieve your balance.)

Put both hands back on the floor in front of you. Come up by reversing the way you went down, straightening the right leg until the knee is locked. Then lower the left foot from the right thigh and shake out the left leg.

Other side: Find your concentration spot on the floor again and, raising the right foot onto the left thigh this time, repeat the posture. Ten seconds. (No Second Set.)

Bikram's Key

If you still can't do this after trying the right way for a few weeks, try this alternate technique: Squat down, put your foot up on the opposite thigh, and only *then* try to balance. Put the fingertips of both hands on the floor, on either side of the body, at first, then try with one hand. Then none.

Benefits

Toe Stand strengthens the knees and is therapeutic for rheumatism of the knees, ankles, and feet. It also opens up the knee and hip joints, and helps cure hemorrhoid problems. As noted earlier, it develops mental strength as well.

Ready for a nice rest? Prepare to enjoy two peaceful minutes of *Savasana*, Dead Body Pose, next in our Sequence. This is the ultimate in rest and relaxation.

Yoga for Obesity and Weight Control

Fat, fat, fat, fat, fat. That's all you hear about these days, and with good reason: Fat is all you see! It's Fat City here, Fat Nation. Fatties "R" Us. You cannot open a newspaper without reading about the growing size of the American body. America has something like 5 percent of the world's population, but I bet if you put everyone in the United States together, they would outweigh the rest of the world!

It's strange: No one in this culture wants to be fat; it's looked down on and considered unattractive. And yet so many of us are so unbelievably fat. It's crazy—a kind of cultural schizophrenia. Beyond that, it's incredibly dangerous as well, probably the biggest health problem we have. You know all the health risks, too, I'm sure. Obesity puts you in danger of developing diabetes, cardiovascular disease, high blood pressure and arthritis, and also can lead to strokes. So why is there so much obesity here and throughout the developed world?

Most people eat three meals a day, and each meal weighs between one and two pounds. As proven by my research at Tokyo University Hospital in the 1970s, an average active person utilizes less than 50 percent of his or her food intake for energy. The other 50 percent remains undigested and is converted to what? FAT. That undigested food gives you a fat ass, a fat face—and a lazy brain, I might add. (Did you think that excess fat was bad for every other part of your body but that it somehow didn't damage your brain's functioning? Don't be ridiculous.)

This unneeded and poorly digested food creates a traffic jam in the body. Circulation is very poor and slow, blood pressure is raised and cholesterol levels go up, too. Victims of this traffic jam will also suffer from heart attacks, varicose veins, phlebitis, coronary thrombosis, pulmonary embolism, adult respiratory disorder syndrome—you name it. Then, before you have begun to properly digest your last meal, you eat again!

Having all this toxic, undigested waste in your system also prevents the nutrition from the food you have managed to digest from being absorbed properly. Too much glucose stays in the bloodstream. So many people—especially in California, where I live—are so fussy about the food they eat, desperately trying to be healthy, and yet their bodies are unable to use even the amazing bounty of delicious and nutritious food available to us here in this country because the organs and systems are not operating and interacting effectively. As I always say: Having something doesn't mean anything if you don't know how to use it.

So what is the best food in the world? *No food*. Don't be scared. I'm not telling you to go on a starvation diet. You will naturally begin to eat less when you consistently practice your yoga. Without dieting or deprivation, your body becomes extremely efficient at processing, transporting and creating fuel. So you eat less, but you absorb your food so much better, and now you're getting the full nutritional benefit. Take me: I eat very little, usually very late. I enjoy food, but I actually *need* to eat very little.

A major American study published in 2005 monitoring weight in over 15,000 people over a 10-year time period showed the power of yoga in weight control. Most people gain a pound a year between the ages of 45 and 55. The average overweight person will gain more, 13.5 pounds, over those same 10 years. In this study those who had a normal weight at age 45 and practiced yoga for four or more years—even for as little as 30 minutes once a week—gained 3 pounds less than the subjects who did no yoga. Imagine what the results would have been if they had practiced 90 minutes of Bikram Yoga every day!

And the overweight people in the study, who had more room for improvement, actually lost 5 pounds, instead of gaining 13.5 as expected.

It's not surprising. Besides improved circulation and a better ability to absorb nutrients, we also know that Hatha Yoga brings a greater awareness of the physical body and a stronger connection with the breath. When you learn to appreciate and then love your body and its awesome capabilities, it's natural that you want to take better care of it. You sense when you are full and stop eating because now you are awake. Plus, the stress hormone cortisol is linked to weight gain—or the inability to lose weight, especially around the abdomen, where accumulation is very dangerous. As discussed in the sidebar on Yoga for Stress (page 111), practicing Hatha Yoga effectively reduces cortisol levels.

Knowing all this doesn't stop me from eating the occasional bacon-wrapped hot dog, however. It tastes good, but I know I'm punishing my body and then I feel bad. Why do I do this, and why do you continue to eat foods that are bad for you, and eat more than you need? Malabsorption keeps you hungry for more, but mainly the reasons are emotional or psychological. Basically, it's greed.

Your body doesn't need all that food you are eating. But your restless, greedy mind that craves simple pleasure and distraction wants it. This is one of the biggest problems we face in life and also one of the greatest benefits that practicing yoga gives us: the ability to distinguish between *want* and *need*. In Part Three of this book I will explain this distinction fully. For now let me just say that when yoga students begin to understand the difference between want and need and are able to act on it, one of the first ways we see it is in their changed relationship to food. The results? Beautiful, slimming changes to their bodies. And on the invisible level, the same liberating changes are happening in their minds. Does that sound good to you, or would you rather keep stuffing your face to fill your fat stomach and serve your screw-loose brain?

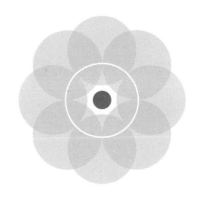

CHAPTER EIGHT

Postures 13-18

Plus: Yoga for Arthritis
and Yoga for Cancer Patients

POSTURE #13:

Dead Body Pose
Savasana

Savasana seems ridiculously simple: Relax and breathe, breathe and relax, while maintaining total stillness. Teaching it takes all of 10 seconds. Yet when properly performed, *Savasana* is the most important posture in Hatha Yoga. Its name translates as "corpse pose," or "dead body pose," due to the complete stillness required during its proper execution (no pun intended). But *Savasana* is actually a powerful way to breathe life into the body. For many people, this is also the most difficult *asana*.

On the physical level, using *Savasana* after certain postures finishes and accelerates the compression and release cycle in which internal organs are first deprived of blood, then flooded with it. Remember our friend Mr. Pancreas? I told you how in certain *asanas* he gets compressed and the blood builds up around him, and then we release the pose and the Hoover Dam breaks— all that oxygenated blood pours in. When this pose is immediately followed by *Savasana*, the circulatory flow is increased to nearly twice its normal speed. The high-speed cleansing flushes out accumulated toxins, free radicals and other debris in its powerful current. This natural irrigation and internal cleansing that occurs after the compression of the postures is how we gain energy through yoga practice. In this way, my class becomes an environmentally friendly gas station for the human body, enabling you to leave more energized and revitalized than when you came in. Without *Savasana*, we discard less waste and receive fewer benefits.

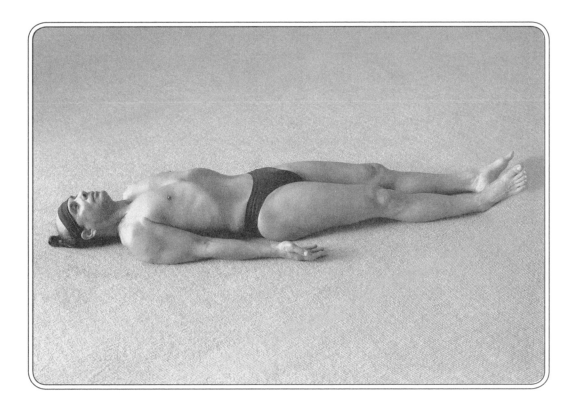

Lying on your back between brief intervals of exercise is a foreign concept to those who exercise by running, jumping or hitting. How many times have you seen someone run half a block, stop, and lie down on the sidewalk for a few moments so their body can adequately absorb the benefits of the exercise? Not many, I'm sure. Forget sports—you don't see this in 99.9 percent of the yoga classes in this country, either. In these diluted styles of Hatha Yoga the students jump around to loud music instead, like in an aerobics class. From a true yogic perspective, this is a crime.

So from here on in the Sequence, we will be performing *Savasana* for a minimum of 20 seconds after each set of every posture.

It goes like this: First Set (which usually means practicing the posture twice; first on one side, then on the other); *Savasana*; Second Set; *Savasana*.

To begin: Lie flat on your back, keeping your limbs straight. Bring your heels together and your arms close enough to almost touch the sides of your body. Turn your palms upward toward the ceiling to release pressure in the shoulder joints, and keep your eyes open to remain present and awake. Relax your whole body as one unit. Let the floor support your full weight.

Concentrate on your breath, inhaling deeply through your nose to the depths of your abdomen up through your chest, and exhaling fully (again, through the nose) from chest to abdomen. Keep the mouth closed. Softly fix your gaze on a single point on the ceiling or an arbitrary point in space. Continue for 2 minutes.

How hard is that; how complicated can it be? Very and very, because now you are dealing with the untrained mind. The mind is rebellious and disobedient. Tell it to do something, and watch it throw a tantrum. When I call for *Savasana* during my classes, I can see the minds of my students begin to mutiny after just 5 or 10 seconds. Toes wiggle, fingers tap, fists and jaws clench, eyes squint, muscles tense, teeth grind and breathing stops. How's that for relaxation? The same things happen when unprepared people attempt sitting meditation. The mind has an agenda of its own, and is terrified of relinquishing control. Submitting to peaceful relaxation will take power away from the ego and its manipulative tools, fear and desire. (I'll explain this dynamic completely in the next section, "Living Yoga.")

But within a few weeks of yoga practice, all the wriggling, fidgeting, clenching, tapping, squinting, waving, holding, locking and grinding in *Savasana* slowly gives way to a peaceful and relaxed stillness. When you are able to make your mind your best friend, *you* have the power, and you achieve a gradual healing and integration of both body and mind.

Bikram's Key

Savasana itself is the only key here, my friend. Go back and read my instructions and relax for 2 full minutes. Enjoy. You can also use this posture at any point in the day or night when you want to relax.

Benefits

Savasana facilitates powerful blood flow, then lets circulation return to normal, creating internal cleansing and greatly magnifying the benefits of the postures that precede it. And in *Savasana* we begin to learn complete relaxation.

POSTURE #14:

Wind-Removing Pose
Pavanamuktasana

Now we move into the floor postures and, in a sense, begin class anew. Because these *asanas* are so powerful and require you to go so deep, we will practice *Savasana* after each set. As its name suggests, Wind-Removing Pose prevents flatulence and it also aids digestion by fighting the production of excess hydrochloric acid. Another deceptively simple-looking pose, it requires full concentration and effort.

To begin: Lying in *Savasana*, bend your right knee up toward your chest. Interlock all ten fingers and grasp that leg just two inches below the knee. Keeping the right foot relaxed, pull the knee down toward your right shoulder slightly, avoiding the rib cage (so you can compress the abdomen). Elbows close to the body. Both shoulders are relaxed, touching the floor.

Keep pulling the knee continuously and smoothly toward your shoulder until you feel a pull in your right hip joint. If you don't feel a strong tug there, you're not pulling hard enough. Tuck your chin into your chest, but don't lift your head up off the floor. The calf of the left leg stays touching the floor; this foot is relaxed, not pointed, please. Every vertebra of your spine is now completely flat on the floor and you should feel pressure in your abdomen. Remember to breathe deeply, and hold this position for 20 seconds.

Lower the right leg back down to the floor, then bend the

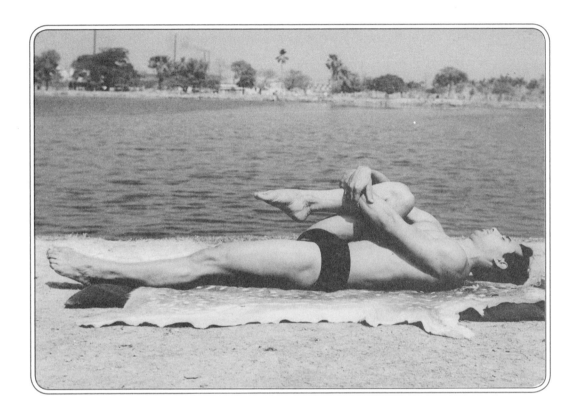

left knee and do the posture on the other side for another 20 seconds.

Next, take hold of both legs and bring them to the chest. Clasp your arms around your legs below your knees and reach your hands across to grab the elbows. If you can't reach, then take hold of the forearms, wrists or fingers—whatever you can reach. Shoulders are down, chin tucked. Try to keep the tailbone and the back of the head touching the floor. Knees are glued together, and glued to the chest. Hold for 20 seconds.

That's one set (with three parts to it). So now we lower the arms and legs to the floor and go into *Savasana* for 20 seconds.

Second Set: Repeat all three parts, then do Dead Body Pose again. You will be more flexible in the Second Set, so pull harder and go deeper. (You will probably be tighter on one side than on the other, as with so many postures.) Push every single vertebra into the floor.

Bikram's Key

To make it easier to get your leg to your chest, try moving the leg a few inches to the side—away from your torso—before pulling it down to the shoulder. It is also essential to keep the calf of the straight leg on the floor. If this gives you difficulty, you can flex the foot toward your face, which will help the calf stay glued to the floor.

Benefits

By pulling the right leg down, you are compressing and massaging the ascending colon. With the left leg, you do the same for the descending colon, and when both legs are glued to the chest you massage the transverse colon and compress the entire digestive system. In addition, this posture strengthens the arms, prevents flatulence, improves hip flexibility, and firms the abdomen and thighs.

Sit-Up

To come out of *Savasana* following Wind-Removing Pose we will do a sit-up. This isn't a posture, but as with *Savasana*, we will be repeating this often during the Sequence. Pay strict attention to my instruction and try to do exactly as I say. Give each sit-up your best, honest effort.

Note: If you have a bad back, I don't recommend you try this. Instead, just roll over onto your front, then gently push yourself up off the ground.

To begin: Lying on the floor, extend both arms overhead and cross your thumbs. *Note:* Do not clasp your hands; just cross the thumbs. Legs are locked, feet flexed back toward your face. Inhale, suck in your stomach, and sit up straight, keeping your arms, head and torso together, legs straight, knees locked, and heels touching the floor.

Don't stop when you are at the 90-degree angle. Instead, start your exhalation and dive forward. As you do, suck in your stomach to activate the core muscles, and as you come down, look at the stomach, bring your chin toward your chest, and curl your torso inward and down (all of this will help create front-side compression). Try to bring the forehead to the knees. Since you are bringing your arms and torso down quickly, with some force behind that action, you'll notice that when you do get your forehead to your knee—or as far down as you are able—you will naturally bounce back up a little bit as the torso rebounds gently upward. Don't try to stop yourself; this actually makes the sit-up safer.

Remember, you exhaled as you came down. Now, at the top of your upward bounce, exhale forcefully again (don't worry about the inhale; that will occur naturally) as you come back down to the curled and folded position. These exhales decrease resistance, compress the abdomen, enhance your acceleration, and relax the body. At the end of this second downward arc, bring the body to rest briefly, ideally with the forehead to the knee, and grabbing your feet or toes with your outstretched fingers. After a pause, get ready to move into your next posture.

Bikram's Key

Make sure you do this in one continuous motion, and don't forget the bounce and double exhale. If you simply can't sit up no matter how hard you try, experiment with lifting the heels and feet a couple of feet in the air before you start the sitting-up motion. Use their added momentum to help you reach your goal.

Benefits

The sit-up strengthens and tones the abdomen, invigorates the body and increases the flexibility of the spine.

Yoga for Arthritis

More than 40 million Americans suffer from osteoarthritis, which is defined as pain and limited motion in the joints. A full third of people in their mid-60s and older have this ailment in just one place: the knee. Unfortunately, this is not just one of the most common medical problems we have here, but also one of the most misunderstood. What is commonly referred to as arthritis is actually not one isolated ailment. It's a component of many related imbalances and pathologies, and the damage it does shows up in a whole other Pandora's box of maladies. What is the cause?

Most Western doctors blame calcium deposits. But how can this be, since calcium is soluble within the human body, and so takes on a liquid form? What exactly is being deposited? Biochemists tell us that the human body produces an excess of acids; one of them is oxalic acid, another liquid. But when oxalic acid is combined with excess calcium they form calcium oxalate, a solid. This calcium oxalate resembles little fish eggs, or caviar, except these fish eggs have sharp edges that traumatize any soft tissue they contact.

These deposits find their home on the tissue they most resemble: bone. However, the bone will only accept such deposits at the joints, where the deposits create the discomfort and loss of mobility that we know as osteoarthritis. (Rheumatoid arthritis, a much less common joint problem, is caused by inflammation, though it can also result in painful deposits, or "nodules," often on the hands and wrists.) This same pathology manifests itself in many ways and goes by many names besides arthritis. Calcium oxalate deposits in the neck or cervical vertebrae, for example, is called spondilitis; in the deltoid joint, frozen shoulder. Then, when that frozen shoulder affects the tendons, you have tendonitis; if it affects the arm, bursitis.

Whatever name you give them, if you do not flush these deposits out of the joints, healing cannot occur. That's where Hatha Yoga comes in. By systematically warming up, moving, twisting, extending and compressing every joint, and putting you into natural human traction, we break down these deposits. (As noted earlier, the debris is then flushed out by the powerful blood flow that results from extension and compression.) I have personally witnessed the radical recovery of thousands of people who were diagnosed as suffering from arthritis in all of its guises. I don't know of a single student who's gotten worse. You don't have to accept this affliction as the unavoidable consequence of growing old. If you practice your Hatha Yoga, your joints, if you can visualize such a thing, will all be wearing smiles.

A study cited in the *Journal of Alternative Complementary Medicine* in 2005 confirms my observations. In the study, people who suffered from osteoarthritis of the knee took very simple Hatha Yoga classes for eight weeks. At the end of the study, a statistically significant number of people had a measurable reduction in pain and disability. Instead of pain medications, then arthroscopic surgery, then incredibly painful knee replacements, all they needed was yoga. My simple remedy for arthritis: Lock the knee!

POSTURE #15:

Cobra Pose
Bhujangasana

Here we begin a series of very important spinal postures. Let me give you a little explanation, so you have a better sense of the scientific thinking underlying this progression. In this posture, Cobra, we will primarily be compressing and strengthening the lower, or lumbar, spine (and of course, all components of the neuromuscular system in that region). The next pose, Locust, focuses on the thoracic spine and some of the cervical spine; then Full Locust focuses more on the upper lumbar and part of the thoracic spine. After that, to use the worst pun in all of yoga, we tie it all together with a bow. What that means is: We complete the four *asanas* of the cobra series by integrating the entire back and spine in the Floor Bow Pose.

After Cobra we will use 80/20 Breathing, creating pneumatic pressure inside the chest and hydraulic pressure in the abdomen to help stabilize and protect the areas being worked here, the torso and spine. Later still, we will build on these and go into even more radical spine-bending, when we do Camel (backward) and Rabbit (forward). Then we will rotate the spine in more of a corkscrew-type motion, while sending increased blood and oxygen to all the spinal nerves, in Spine-Twisting Pose, the very last *asana*.

So we're addressing the spine systematically: first with poses for the lower, upper and middle sections, then with an integrated posture, and finally with even deeper motions, backward and forward. Why do we give the spine all this rigorous and loving at-

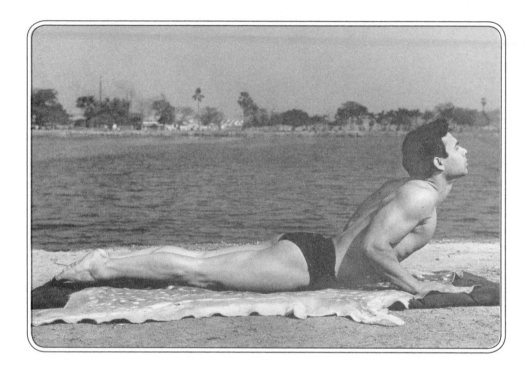

tention? Because as I said before (quoting my guru), the spine is the source of all energy, the center of our human body's life. So a healthy spine equals a healthy life.

To begin: Lie on your stomach, legs and feet together. Tighten the muscles in your legs and hip area, including the glutes, lock your knees, and point your toes. Place your palms on the floor, fingertips under the tops of your shoulders, fingers pointing forward. Elbows are in, touching your sides.

Look up at the ceiling, raise your head, and, using the strength of your back, lift your torso off the floor. Arch the head and torso back as much as possible; at the same time, press the belly button into the floor. The belly button and everything below it stays in contact with the floor. As a beginner you may not be strong enough to do this with your spine and back muscles alone; you need help. In that case, use your arm strength to push your torso higher. In the future, you won't need your arms to lift yourself, but for now it's okay.

Your elbows should be bent at 90-degree angles, tight to your sides. The shoulders are relaxed and down. Stay arched for 20 seconds, then slowly lower yourself back to the floor. Turn your face to one side, arms down at your sides, and relax on your stomach for 20 seconds. This is also *Savasana*, even though we are lying facedown instead of faceup as we practiced it before. After all the postures done in the spinal/Cobra series we will rest in *Savasana* this way. As always, keep your eyes open.

Second Set: Repeat the posture for 20 seconds and then relax again for 20 seconds.

Bikram's Key

This is one of the most difficult postures to learn and to understand. So we need two keys here. First, when you finish holding the arched position, don't suddenly collapse back down to the floor. Lower your head, neck and upper body slowly and smoothly, using the strength of your back and spine. We never use any abrupt diving or jerking motions; that's how you injure yourself. Controlling your movements this way also builds will power and discipline.

Second, keep your elbows close to the ribs. As you come up, try to slide them down toward the hip bones, as if you were going to touch them with the elbow points. This moves your shoulders and keeps them down, where they belong. The trapezius muscles—the sheets of muscle just under the skin of the back, between the shoulders and neck—should protrude and become more visible.

Benefits

Cobra strengthens the lumbar spine, relieving pain and combating slipped or herniated discs, scoliosis and arthritis in that region. But it is also one of the best all-around conditioners we have for the entire body. Other important benefits include improved digestion, relief from menstrual disorders, improved appetite, and raising low blood pressure. Cobra also improves the functioning of the liver and spleen and strengthens the deltoids, trapezius, and triceps muscles in the upper body.

POSTURE #16:

Locust Pose
Salabhasana

Locust Pose is made up of three components, and the last stage is probably the most hated part of my entire class. Many students simply cannot lift both legs off the floor together, or hold them there for more than a few seconds, and that can be incredibly frustrating. Patience. Stay strong, do your best, and this last part of Locust will soon be a piece of cheesecake. Well, maybe not that easy.

To begin: Lie on your stomach, with your chin resting on the floor. Here's the tricky part: Place your arms under your body with your elbows turned up against the abdomen and palms flat on the floor, fingers spread and pointing toward your feet, little fingers side by side. Both arms are pinned under your body. Feet together. The best news I can give you is: Your elbows will only hurt for a week or so after you begin this practice.

Now raise the right leg, keeping it straight with the knee locked, to a 45-degree angle with the floor. Don't lift all the way up to the hip; the right hip should stay down. Don't rotate, twist or bend the leg in any way, shape or fashion. That knee is locked. Hold the right leg up for 10 seconds.

Slowly lower the right leg to the floor. Maintaining the same straitjacketed position of your body and arms, lift the left leg up to a 45-degree angle—don't twist the leg or lift the hip. If you hold your foot in what feels like a slightly pigeon-toed position,

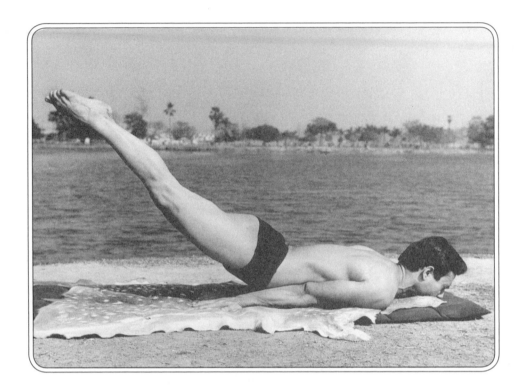

you will actually be doing this right. Keep the leg raised for another 10 full seconds.

Slowly lower the left leg. Release your head and chin so you
are now facedown, with no bend in the neck. Your arms are still
trapped. Now lock both knees, point your toes, and tense your
thigh and hip muscles until they are hard as rocks. Squeeze your
legs together, take a big inhale, and raise *both* of your legs—and
the hips, this time—off the floor as high as possible.

Begin 80/20 Breathing and hold the pose for 10 seconds.

After the 10 count, lower both legs slowly, under control,
knees locked. Again, lowering the legs smoothly builds back,
core and spinal strength. Pull your arms out from under the body

and relax them at your sides, palms up. Turn your face to one side and relax on your stomach with your eyes open for 20 seconds.

Second Set: Repeat each part of the pose for 10 seconds. Then relax facedown for another 20 seconds, eyes open.

Bikram's Key

In all three phases of Locust, reaching and stretching your legs *out*, away from your body, is the important thing, not how high you lift them. (And, as always, your knees must be locked.) Imagine that someone has hooked your big toe to one of my Bentleys and I'm driving it through the wall behind you.

In the last, most hated part of Locust—lifting both legs at once—understand that you're not really doing this with the legs on their own. When you can accomplish this lift, it will be because the muscles of the lower back and abdomen are doing the work; *they're* picking up the legs and moving them. So if you're struggling here, send mental messages to those areas, and to your lower spine, telling them to send more power right away!

Benefits

The Locust pose has many of the same benefits as Cobra, but it is even better for slipped discs and sciatica. It strengthens the upper spine, and the uncomfortable stretching of the arms can actually relieve tennis elbow. Locust can also help with varicose veins in the legs.

POSTURE #17:

Full Locust Pose
Poorna-Salabhasana

Here we focus on the mid-spine, combining the action in Cobra (lifting the upper body) with that of Locust (in which you raised the legs). With nothing to prop you up, no limbs to push with, you want to end up perfectly balanced on your hip bones. We will use 80/20 Breathing once we achieve the pose.

To begin: Lying on your stomach, extend both arms out to the sides, palms down. As in Locust, raise your head and rest your chin on the floor. Keeping your legs together, point your toes, lock both knees, and tighten all the muscles in the legs and hip area. Keeping them tensed will prevent you from letting your knees or feet fly apart when you finally get into this "airplane" pose.

Start with a big inhale, raise your head and chin off the floor to look at the ceiling, and in one movement raise both arms, both legs and your entire torso off the floor. Your arms are now lifting up and moving backward slightly, looking like the wings on your personal Concorde jet. Your palms face the floor, fingers together. The fingertips should be level with the top of your head, palms parallel to the floor.

Begin 80/20 Breathing. Ideally you will use the muscles of the middle and lower spine to remain perfectly balanced on the hip bones for 10 honest seconds.

Come down slowly. Turn your head to one side, arms relaxed at your sides, and rest facedown for 20 seconds in *Savasana.*

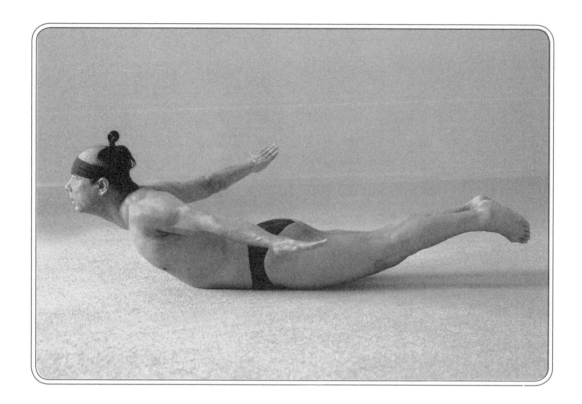

Second Set: Do Full Locust again for another 10 seconds, then rest for another 20.

Bikram's Key

Of all the postures in the Hatha Yoga, this one is the most difficult to improve in. Even after five years, you may only get your torso and arms to come up 1 inch higher. But that's okay—if you're trying the right way, the benefit is still amazing. You can sacrifice height in raising the legs in favor of raising the front of the body. Concentrate on that. Try to raise the legs but know it's okay if they lag behind.

Benefits

Full Locust increases strength in the middle spine; it is good for scoliosis, kyphosis, spondylosis and slipped discs. Like the Standing Bow pose, it opens up the rib cage and increases elasticity there. It also firms the abdominal muscles, upper arms, hips and thighs.

POSTURE #18:

Bow Pose
Dhanurasana

All the postures you've done so far have prepared you nicely to do one good Bow posture. As the spine is the source of energy in the human body, integrating the spine leads to a balanced, healthy body, and a balanced, healthy and successful life. Bow Pose will show you where you are inflexible and where your mind still has trouble connecting with your body. (Surfers, who have strong lower backs, are often great at this pose and Full Locust right away.) The other good news is that while Bow Pose combines all the challenges of Cobra, Locust, Full Locust, Standing Bow and Balancing Stick, it also combines all their fantastic benefits.

To begin: Lie on your stomach. Bend your knees behind you and then lower your heels down toward your hips. Reach backward and take hold of both insteps from the outside, keeping all five fingers together, about 2 inches below the toes. Get a firm grip; you will need it.

Inhale deeply, look up at the ceiling, point your toes, and lift your thighs off the floor; doing this will lift the upper body as well. Begin 80/20 Breathing.

As in the Standing Bow we did much earlier, kicking backward and upward against your hands will lift the legs even higher off the floor. As your legs move higher, roll forward, moving your body weight and your center of gravity until you are balanced on

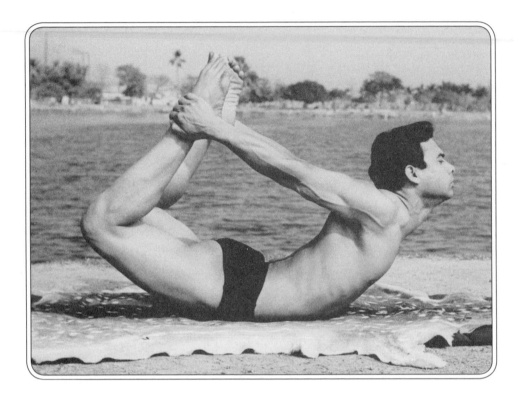

the center of your abdomen. Everyone has a different spinal structure so this will look slightly different for each person. But the principle is the same. Stay motionless in the pose for 20 seconds.

It's very important to come out of this intense pose slowly and with control. Lower the torso and legs deliberately and then relax for 20 seconds, facedown with your head turned to the side in *Savasana*.

Second Set: Repeat the posture for 20 seconds, then rest for another 20 seconds.

Bikram's Key

Don't pull with the arms—just kick up with the legs. That's what lifts your upper body. In the beginning your legs will splay outward; keep them, and your feet, just 6 inches apart.

Benefits

You'll feel instantly how Bow Pose opens up the rib cage, which allows the lungs to expand more fully. This 360-degree flexion of the spine revitalizes all the spinal nerves by increasing circulation, and strengthens the spine along its entire length. Besides helping with all manner of back problems, Bow aids digestion, fights constipation, and combats bronchitis and diabetes while improving the functioning of the large and small intestines, the liver, kidneys and spleen. It also stretches and strengthens the abdominal wall.

Yoga for Cancer Patients

Based on decades of personal observation, I know that Hatha Yoga prevents and successfully fights many forms of cancer. But I understand that the American public only wants to hear the "proof," what the Western medical establishment says is clinically shown to be true. So I will confine myself here to what is "proven" in that way. So far, what has been shown most clearly has to do with yoga benefiting cancer patients in their recovery, rather than preventing or curing the disease itself.

Some of the best evidence relates to breast cancer patients. As you probably know, this disease is extremely common and widespread; one in eight women in North America will be diagnosed with breast cancer. The allopathic Western treatments used, from radical surgery and mastectomy to radiation and chemotherapy, are brutal and painful, with physical side effects such as nausea and fatigue, and emotional ones that include depression and anxiety.

In work done by Dr. Alyson Moadel at the Albert Einstein College of Medicine in the Bronx, New York, 126 women who were taking chemotherapy did 12 weeks of gentle *asanas* and *pranayama* and used tapes to practice at home daily. The breathing exercises helped tremendously with the nausea, and the women who practiced yoga were less tired and had better overall physical functioning than those in the a control group, who did not practice yoga. On the emotional or spiritual side, the women who practiced Hatha Yoga said it helped them to deal better with their illness. They felt better, with less depression and less anxiety. (If yoga can do that for women with a life-threatening disease, imagine how much better you can feel if you are lucky enough to be cancer-free!)

These positive results have also been seen in research at the M.D. Anderson Cancer Center at the University of Texas, and the physical and emotional benefits of yoga are now being studied in regard to other forms of cancer as well. Experience tells me that the same benefits will be seen. In fact, in a surprising sign of medical sanity, it was recently reported that up to 10 percent of all women undergoing cancer treatment (for any kind of cancer) are doing some form of therapeutic yoga as part of their care. That number should be 100 percent, but it's a start.

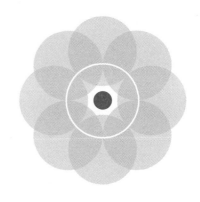

CHAPTER NINE

Postures 19-26
Second Breathing
Exercise

Plus: Yoga for Diabetes

POSTURE #19:

Fixed Firm Pose
Supta-Vajrasana

Because of the compression of the knees, this Fixed Firm Pose can be difficult for athletes and big men. But it will also radically improve the physiology of the knees, ankles and hips of those who practice it with dedication and determination.

To begin: Sit down with your buttocks on your heels, knees and feet together as they do in Japan. (While I was teaching there I learned that they call this position *seiza.*) Now, keeping the knees together, move the feet hip-width apart, so that you're sitting down on the floor between your feet. Soles are facing up and the sides of your feet are pointing straight back behind you, hugging the sides of the hips.

Reach behind you and place the palms of your hands on your upturned toes, thumbs inside, fingers pointing forward. Holding on to your feet, slowly bend your right elbow down to the floor behind you, then bend the left elbow and bring it to the floor, so that your torso is now leaning backward supported by the elbows. Do this s-l-o-w-l-y. Keeping your knees touching the floor—and touching each other—let your head drop back, and then your shoulders and torso, slowly lowering them all to the floor.

After the upper back is down, slide the elbows out from under you. Now raise your arms up over your head and lay them flat on the floor, elbows bent and hands clasping the opposite elbows. Tuck your chin into your chest. Stay here for 20 seconds.

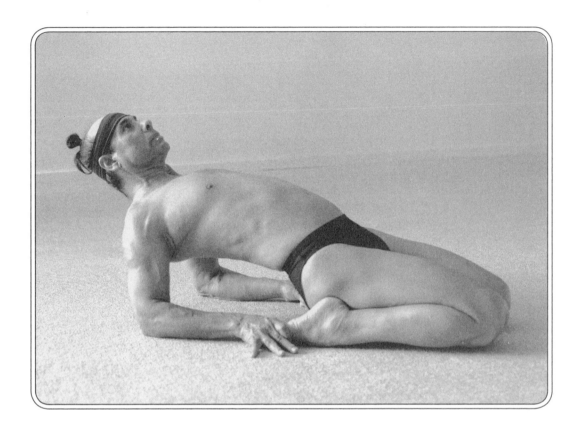

Use your elbows and hands to help yourself come up slowly, the same way you went in. Rest in *Savasana* for 20 seconds.

Next, do a sit-up, taking hold of the toes and touching your forehead to your knees. Don't forget to bounce twice.

Second Set: Repeat Fixed Firm for another 20 seconds, then rest in *Savasana* for 20 more seconds.

Bikram's Key

If you can't do this or have too much pain performing the posture this way, you can separate the knees before lowering the elbows. When you don't need to do that anymore, focus on keeping your knees touching and flat on the floor.

Benefits

Fixed Firm Pose strengthens and improves the flexibility of the lower spine, hips, knees and ankle joints. It increases circulation to the lower limbs, and is therapeutic for lower back pain, sciatica, rheumatism and varicose veins. It also strengthens the psoas muscles and helps prevent hernias. It's beneficial for the spleen—the filter for the lymphatic system—which helps the liver as well as strengthening the entire immune system.

POSTURE #20:

Half Tortoise Pose
Ardha-Kurmasana

By training us to slow our breathing and relax, Half Tortoise Pose can actually help us to live longer—in fact, longevity is Tortoise's number one benefit. Think about it: The tortoise is the longest-living animal on Earth. There's one in the Calcutta Zoo that's 550 years old! Why? Because it's the *slowest-breathing* creature on Earth. Each inhale and each exhale is 2 minutes long; it's like a meditation in itself. We do ourselves good when we imitate the Tortoise; 30 seconds in this posture can provide the same benefits to the body as sleeping for a full eight hours. You can get this restorative, relaxing effect by practicing Tortoise at any time, even in bed.

To begin: Sit on your heels, knees and feet together. Raise and straighten your arms overhead, lock your elbows, and place the palms together, crossing the thumbs. Reach your arms up as high as you can and inhale fully. On the exhale, suck in your stomach and bend forward slowly, keeping your body in one straight line from tailbone to fingertips, until the edges of your little fingers touch the floor. At the same time, bring your forehead to the floor and rest it there. Keep your hips down on your heels; don't lift the body off them. Your elbows are locked, wrists and arms straight, eyes open.

Reach forward even more with your arms. Stay here for 20 seconds, breathing deeply.

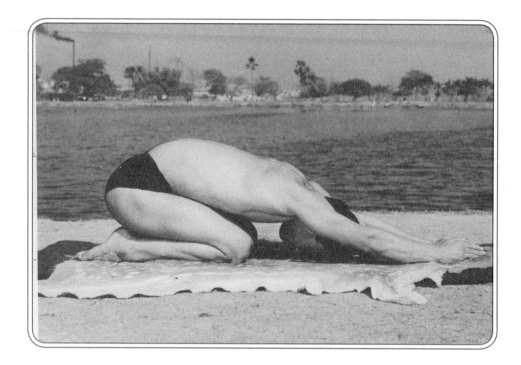

Come up exactly as you went down—lifting slowly and in one piece, stomach sucked in, back straight. One straight line. Then turn over and rest in *Savasana* for 20 seconds. Do another perfect sit-up, then kneel again.

Second Set: Repeat the posture for 20 seconds, then rest in *Savasana* for 20 seconds.

Bikram's Key

To accomplish this posture without sagging and breaking the straight line of your arms and upper body, you'll need to generate a tremendous amount of power in your hands and arms and especially the muscles in your abdomen, back and sides. You'll feel how much you are working the core and strengthening the spine. If you have tight hips or a big stomach, this can be quite hard. Don't be discouraged.

Benefits

Aside from enhancing longevity, Tortoise is great for tense necks and shoulders. It also increases blood flow to the brain, which enhances memory and mental clarity. This posture also stretches the lower part of the lungs, which is therapeutic for asthma, and counters indigestion, flatulence, constipation and irritable bowel syndrome. Plus, it increases flexibility of the hip joints. Got a headache? Do two Half Tortoise poses and call me in the morning.

Yoga for Diabetes

In yoga we say that diabetes is essentially a bad marriage between the pancreas and the kidneys. However, in Western medical terms we can't "prove" this yet; one day we'll know for sure!

Everyone agrees that the pancreas is supposed to produce insulin, the hormone that allows us to absorb glucose, or blood sugar—the energy we need to live—from our food. When it doesn't supply enough of this juice, high blood pressure, anemia (due to the kidneys' inability to produce enough red blood cells) and even outright kidney failure can occur. Not having enough insulin causes Type 1 diabetes.

In the much more common Type 2 diabetes, the body cannot properly absorb insulin; these people are "insulin resistant." In either of these bad-news scenarios, severe damage to the heart, brain, eyes or legs—as well as the kidneys—can result. Other symptoms of diabetes include memory loss, peripheral neuropathy and, for men, impotence.

Diabetes now affects roughly *18 million people* in the United States. Obesity, especially fat around the abdomen, is a major risk factor for Type 2 diabetes, and diabetics who are obese are in turn at higher risk for coronary artery disease and strokes. Did you know that diabetes is now the fifth leading cause of death in this country? As if that's not scary enough, this pandemic has spread to American children, generations of our kids who are not just overweight but at risk for their very lives.

Giving yourself an insulin injection may alleviate the symptoms of diabetes for a while, but it is not a cure. It does not solve the problem of the bad marriage between your pancreas and kidneys. For years, yogis have claimed better blood-sugar balance comes from regular Hatha Yoga practice, and recent studies at the University College of Medical Sciences in New Delhi and the Bhabha Research Centre in Mumbai indeed found that performing postures regularly decreased blood-sugar levels. Yoga also had a slimming effect, quantified in the study as "decreased hip-to-waist ratios," which also helped to normalize insulin levels. As the study noted in its conclusion: "Yoga *asanas* may be used as an excellent adjunct with diet and drugs in management of Type 2 Diabetes."

Bow and Rabbit postures, because of the way they compress the kidneys and pancreas, respectively, are especially therapeutic. But the best prescription for diabetes is doing the entire Sequence, every day. My student Julian wrote a book about how yoga controlled his diabetic symptoms, which came on when he was only 27 years old. He suffered until he was 54, when he came to me. "I thought I would die from that first yoga class," he writes. But he didn't give up; for one thing, he'd paid for a year's worth of classes. What happened? After six months, he no longer needed the medicine he'd been taking for decades. (He also lost 50 pounds without dieting and cleared up his chronic back problem.) The title of his book is *Diabetic Always*, but the subtitle is *Insulin No More!*

POSTURE #21:

Camel Pose
Ustrasana

Okay, now we are going into the deepest backbend of all. If you tried this at the beginning of class, you wouldn't be prepared; your spine wouldn't be warmed up enough and you'd injure yourself. But at this point we've warmed up the body and the spine for 75 or 80 minutes. Despite the extreme bend in Camel, we don't need to use 80/20 Breathing because, unlike the backbend in Half Moon, where you are standing unsupported, or the one in Bow, where you are working against gravity, here you are kneeling and stabilized on the floor.

This is one of the most powerful, important postures of all, along with *Savasana*, Rabbit, and the Spinal Twisting pose. Camel may even be slightly ahead of the last two, because of how well it compensates for all the chair-sitting and leaning and bending forward we do in our daily lives.

To begin: Stand up straight on your knees this time, rather than sitting on your heels. Your knees and feet are 6 inches apart. (If you find it very uncomfortable to keep your knees only 6 inches apart, you may move them slightly farther away from each other. But the feet must remain just 6 inches apart throughout.)

Put your hands on the backs of your hips, fingers pointing down, thumbs to the outside. The hands will support your lower back. Keeping your hands on your hips, take a deep breath in, hold it, then drop your head backward. Slowly bend the entire

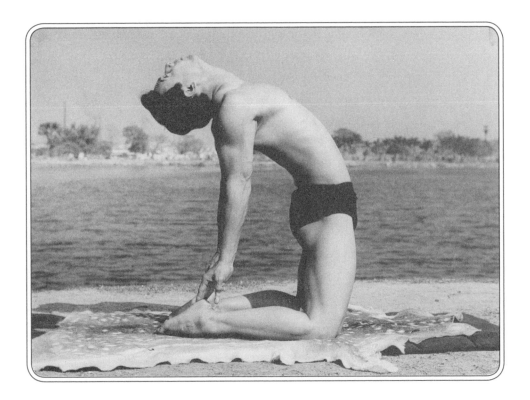

torso backward as far as you can go. At the same time, you will naturally exhale. Now slowly and carefully reach your right hand down, taking hold of your right heel. Your thumb should be to the outside of the foot. Then do the same with the left hand, taking hold of the left heel. If you can't grab your heels at first, keep the hands on the backs of the hips, supporting the back.

Take a deep inhale, then exhale strongly as you push your thighs, hips and stomach forward as much as possible. This will arch your torso backward—Newton's Third Law in action again. You will definitely feel this throughout your entire back and spine. Hold the position for 20 seconds.

Come up by reversing the way you went down: Slowly take

the right hand off the right heel and place it back on the right hip, then do the same with the left hand. Then lie down for 20 seconds of *Savasana*.

Take a deep inhale, then do a perfect sit-up.

Second Set: Repeat Camel for 20 seconds, then rest in *Savasana* for 20 seconds.

Bikram's Key

There's no pulling on the heels. You're just holding them. All the power in this posture comes from exhaling and pushing the midsection forward. Concentrate on the area from the top of your thighs to your chest, and on pushing it up and forward with all the strength in your muscles and spine. This area will actually stretch and expand with accordion-like elasticity.

Benefits

Camel Pose creates maximum compression of the spine, which stimulates the nervous system. It also improves flexibility of the neck and spine, relieves backache, and helps degenerative spinal problems such as kyphoscoliotic deformities and cervical spondylosis. By stretching the abdominal organs, Camel helps constipation, and it also stretches the throat and thyroid and parathyroid glands.

Like Bow Pose, it opens narrow rib cages to give more space to the lungs. Camel also firms and slims the abdomen and the waistline.

POSTURE #22:

Rabbit Pose
Sasangasana

Rabbit Pose is the most radical forward-bending and spinal compression in the Sequence. The object of the pose is to stretch out the spine slowly, as though all the vertebrae were a pearl necklace on an elastic string. In the stretch we nourish and align everything on that string, and then, when the tension is slowly released, all the pearls come back together and the integrity of the spine is restored. You may feel afterward that your spine is literally longer than when you began. Such is the power of this posture that you may actually be right.

To begin: Sit down on your heels Japanese-style, with your knees and feet together. Reach back behind you and grab your heels with either hand, palms down, with the thumbs on the outside of the feet, fingers to the inside. (You can improve your grip around the heels by wrapping the edges of your towel over the heels, and grasping both together.) Now you're cupping your heels in your palms, gripping them tightly.

Look at your stomach, lower your chin to your chest, and, on an exhale, curl your torso forward slowly until your forehead is touching your knees and the top of your head is touching the floor. Once the top of your head is touching the floor, lift your hips into the air. Pulling on your heels with all your strength, straighten your arms completely. As your body rolls forward, your thighs will move also, until they are perpendicular to the floor. You want the tension between your arms and heels to hold up

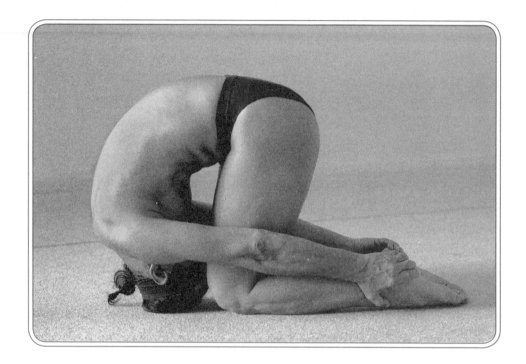

most of your weight, instead of resting that weight on your head
and neck. A maximum of 25 percent of your weight should be on
your head. Because of the tucked chin, you may feel a little
choked in your throat. Ignore that—welcome it, even. You're
massaging your thyroid and compressing the throat, which also
massages the lymph nodes.

Stay here for 20 seconds, with your eyes on your stomach.
Keep the stomach sucked in to provide compression.

Still holding your heels, reverse the forward curl and slowly
come back to the kneeling position. Relax on your back in *Savasana* for 20 seconds. Do a sit-up, then kneel.

Second Set: Repeat Rabbit Pose for 20 seconds. Follow it with another 20 seconds of *Savasana*.

Bikram's Key

The secret here is in the arms: You must pull with all your strength on the heels of both feet to perform the posture fully and to keep your weight where it belongs.

If you can't touch the forehead to the knees, walk the knees up, one by one, to the forehead. Don't relax the grip or your arms. *Note:* Never move your head while in the completed posture, to prevent injury to your cervical spine and neck.

Benefits

Maximum extension of the spine increases its mobility and elasticity, and does the same for the back muscles. Spinal stretching also expedites the feeding of the nervous system with fresh blood and oxygen. Rabbit Pose relieves tension in the neck, shoulders and back. It helps alleviate colds, sinus problems, and chronic tonsillitis and, through compression of thyroid and para-thyroid, rejuvenates those glands as well. Rabbit Pose can also be therapeutic for insomnia, diabetes and depression.

POSTURES #23 AND #24:

Head to Knee Pose and Stretching Pose

Janushirasana and *Paschimotthanasana*

This combination of poses creates a wonderful stretch in the sciatic nerves, which helps prevent and treat that common and painful condition, sciatica. It also improves the flexibility of the last five vertebrae of the spine, as well as the ankle, knee, hip, shoulder, elbow and wrist joints. When you stretch out over one extended leg in the first two parts of this Sequence, you will once again find that one side is more flexible than the other. As I said before, this just proves that you are human.

To begin: Sitting on the floor or on a mat, stretch your left leg out diagonally so that your two legs form a 90-degree angle. Bend your right knee and bring your right heel into the groin area near the top of your right leg. Lock the right knee.

Raise both arms overhead and interlock your fingers. Tuck your chin into your chest and bend down over the outstretched leg. Move the arms and mid-body as one unit. Grasp the left foot firmly in both hands, with the fingers interlocked beneath the ball of the foot and the toes. The thumbs stay crossed under the toes. Try to lock the left knee, then bring the forehead to the knee. Beginners may have to bend the leg to bring the forehead to the knee. Press down with your forehead on the knee, keeping the grip on the foot and toes. Eventually, doing this will allow you to lock the knee.

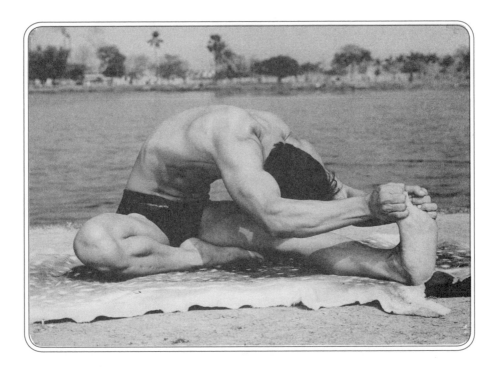

Either way, pull the toes back toward you, with your chin tucked. Bend your elbows and bring them down to the floor. Bring your left elbow, shoulder and knee down closer to the floor by rolling your body slightly to the left of your outstretched leg. Stay here for 10 seconds.

Come up slowly, and then reverse the pose with the right leg extended, left leg bent. Use the same rolling action to bring your left elbow closer to the floor. Hold for 10 seconds. Then come up slowly and extend both legs straight out in front of you. Now we're ready for *Paschimotthanasana*, Stretching Pose.

Raise both arms overhead, thumbs crossed, and recline backward to the floor. As soon as you touch, inhale deeply and do an immediate sit-up. Take hold of your big toes with the first two fingers of each hand, palms facing each other. Pull the toes

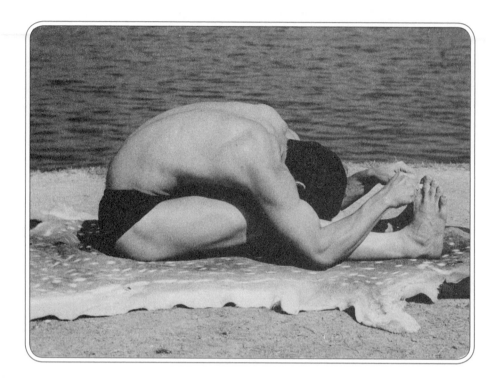

toward you as much as possible. Wiggle your hips backward right and left a few times; that will help you reach forward a little farther. Try to lock both knees. If your knees are locked with the thighs tightly contracted, then lower your stomach to your thighs. If your knees stay locked, then lower your chest to your knees, keeping your back as flat as possible, chin up.

Now bend both elbows and try to pull your heels up off the floor. Eventually, you will be able to touch your forehead to your knees. Keep your knees locked, thighs tight. Stay here 20 seconds.

Come up slowly, then rest in *Savasana* for 20 seconds. Bring yourself back up with a sit-up.

Second Set: Repeat Head to Knee Pose for 10 seconds on each side and Stretching Pose for 20 seconds. Then rest again for 20 seconds.

Bikram's Key

As a beginner, you may not be able to lock your knees. No problem. Pull on the toes, and try to straighten your legs on the floor, chest up, back flat. If you feel a pull in the backs of your knees and legs, that's good. That means you are stretching the sciatic nerves, thigh biceps and calf muscles.

Benefits

Besides all the stretching I describe above, the combination of Head to Knee Pose and Stretching Pose is also excellent for the immune and lymphatic systems, and increases circulation to the liver, spleen, pancreas, thyroid, thymus and intestines. It improves digestion and is good for allergies and arthritis. Stretching Pose also relieves chronic diarrhea by improving the circulation in the bowels.

POSTURE #25

Spine-Twisting Pose
Ardha-Matsyendrasana

Now that every part of the body, including all areas of the spine, is flexed and warm, we can perform this very powerful manipulation, the spinal twist.

To begin: In a seated position, place the side of the right knee on the floor and bring your right heel to touch the outside of your left hip. Now lift the left leg in the air, bringing it over the bent right leg, and place your left foot just to the outside of the right knee. This leg is bent at the knee, sole of the foot flat on the floor. Touch the outside corner of the right knee with your left heel.

Bring your right arm up and over to the left, then bring it down on the outside of your left knee, with the elbow pressing back against it. Take hold of the right knee with your right hand, grasping the kneecap firmly. (If you can't reach the right knee, just keep pressure against the left knee with the elbow.)

Now put your left arm behind your back, palm facing out, and reach all the way around your body until you can touch or grasp the right thigh. In this way, we begin the twist. You may not be able to reach the thigh at this point; if not, simply place the left hand down on the floor behind you and use it to support your body, keeping it upright.

Turn your head to the left and rotate your face, shoulders and torso to the left, twisting as much as possible. It is important to try to keep both buttocks and the right knee on the floor, and

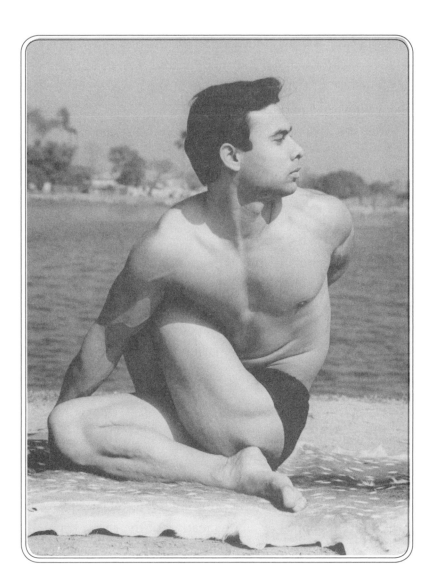

maintain a straight spine. Here, fully emptying the lungs in Normal Breathing facilitates the twist. As you exhale, try to twist around a little farther. Hold the posture for 20 seconds.

Unwind slowly, then reverse the legs and arms, and do the pose for 20 seconds on the other side. Here's another technique that will help you twist farther: Before you turn, lift your upper body toward the ceiling, and try to lift the abdomen up and out of the pelvis, so you can twist more of the torso, including the abdomen when you turn.

After you've done the second side, rest in *Savasana* for 20 seconds.

Note: We do this posture only once.

Bikram's Key

First, make sure the heel of the foot is touching the knee, not higher up on the thigh. Second, when you bring your arm over and across, place the hand so it, the knee and the heel are all touching at the same spot. Third, point the toes of the leg bent on the floor, heel touching the outside of the hip.

Benefits

This is the only posture that twists the spine from top to bottom, which increases circulation to all the spinal nerves, veins, and tissues, and improves the elasticity of the spine (it also helps open the hip joints). Spine Twisting relieves lower back pain and helps prevent slipped discs, rheumatism of the spine, kyphosis, scoliosis, cervical spondylosis and arthritis. It also calms the nervous system.

SECOND BREATHING EXERCISE AND POSTURE #26:

Blowing in Firm Pose
Kapalbhati in *Vajrasana*

As you perform this combination of the second breathing exercise and the last *asana* in my Sequence—your last bit of self-improvement before relaxing in final *Savasana*—you will be improving digestion and circulation, and increasing the elasticity of the lungs with every forceful exhale. You generate *prana*, and push out every ounce of carbon dioxide, replacing it with life-giving oxygen.

To begin: Kneel down Japanese-style, sitting on your heels, hands on your knees, elbows locked. Sit up straight. Begin to blow out your breath powerfully through your pursed, open lips— as if you were blowing out a candle 20 feet in front of you. Just exhale repeatedly; the inhales will occur naturally.

As you exhale, pull in the stomach vigorously. This expels the air. When it's in and the exhale is finished, relaxing the stomach muscles creates the inhale. Then pull the abdomen in again— moving your belly button toward the back of your spine—with the next exhale. Only the stomach moves, nothing else. Not the head, not the shoulders, the arms, or the lower back.

Continue this breathing cycle, maintaining the force of the exhales. Do this at least 60 times. Rest for several seconds, still sitting Japanese-style.

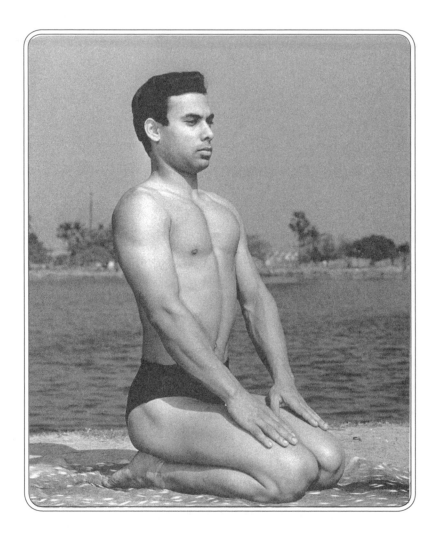

Second Set: Do the exercise again for another 60 breaths, exhaling more rapidly than in the first set. Now lie down and rest in *Savasana* for as long as you like.

Bikram's Key

This vigorous movement of the stomach takes practice to perform properly. To accelerate your progress, try placing a hand on the abdomen, on or around the navel, as you begin your exhalations. This way you can tell immediately if the midsection is moving inward as it should. An alternate method is to start by pushing the stomach *outward*, letting it hang out completely relaxed, which will exaggerate and accelerate the inward motion when it comes.

Benefits

Besides the benefits to the lungs described above, *Kapalbhati* also strengthens the abdominal organs and increases circulation to them. Blowing in Firm stimulates the digestive system as well.

Congratulations! Class is over and you've made it through. Even if this was your first-ever class, your body is absorbing the effects of the practice and beginning to change—refreshing, revitalizing and reorganizing itself in every cell and molecule.

In some ways, the beginning class you've just been through is all there is to my teachings, and to the way of yoga. On a foundational level I have only one essential message, requirement, or recommendation: *Practice Hatha Yoga*. Every day. That's all you need to do. (If some days you are traveling or have less time, you can do a Half Class, simply performing each *asana* once instead of twice. No Second Sets.)

On the next level the 26 postures and two breathing exercises are just the beginning. In the rest of this book I will describe all the wonderful changes that you can now expect—the fantastic, life-altering results of your yoga practice. I'll teach you, as I was taught, the lessons the great yogis and the Indian tradition offer us for living our lives outside the classroom or studio. To the yoga of the body we will add the yoga of the mind and, finally, the yoga of life. I offer all this to you joyfully, to give guidance and purpose to your journey and bring fulfillment to your Soul.

PART THREE

Living Yoga

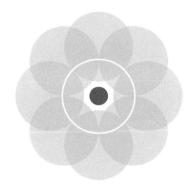

Once you have trained the body through the physical practice of Hatha Yoga, you can begin to control the mind, making your current Number One Enemy into your new best friend. We'll learn how the mind works—including where it goes astray—and the essential qualities of mind a yogi must have. I will provide practical suggestions and exercises to develop those mental qualities and replace bad habits with good ones.

To reach Self-Realization, we must fulfill the requirements of our Karma Yoga, through the practice of Hatha Yoga (the body) and Raja Yoga (the mind). After you've improved both your body and your mind, the Spirit will reenter or reawaken in your beautified temple. This puts you on the path to realize your true destiny, the realization of the godly potential we all have inside. That's our ultimate goal.

Once you are on this path, my friend, your life will necessarily be much different—you're not the same person anymore. You will need a new map to the rest of your life, and I will provide that in the pages that follow. I'll reveal how yoga tells us how we should live, including the Four Stages, or steps, in one lifetime and what karmic duties we must perform in each of them to gain true happiness on this Earth. Among these teachings will be guidance on love and marriage and the importance of faith (not organized religion), which is the basis of Spirituality.

To these traditional ideas I will add my observations, not just from my 50-plus years practicing yoga but also from my 35 years in the United States, showing you how you can combine ancient Indian wisdom with current American know-how, opportunity and advancements to create the best life possible.

Once again, there is no easy way. The only way is the right way, and the right way is the hard way. With my guidance and encouragement and your supreme effort, you can become your own guru and *lead yourself* to that ideal existence, the best of both worlds.

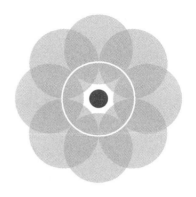

CHAPTER TEN

Mastering
the Mind

Yoga is a method for restraining the natural turbulence of thoughts, which otherwise impartially prevents all men, of all lands, from glimpsing their true nature of Spirit. So long as man possesses a mind with its restless thoughts, so long will there be a universal need for yoga.

—*Paramahansa Yogananda*

DID YOU KNOW THAT YOU OWN A FERRARI? OR, SINCE PEOPLE are different from one another, maybe you have a Lamborghini instead. Either way, it is a world-class car, so powerful it can exceed 200 mph. Unless, of course, the battery terminal has a loose connection, in which case the car won't move. All it takes is one tiny part to fail before the car breaks down.

The human body—your beautiful car—is the same way. If one little part of the body doesn't work, you collapse. It doesn't have to be a big thing. Something small like a cold or the flu, stomach cramps, gas, or a little headache will keep your machine from functioning the way it was built to. If you have illness, my guru said, all your appointments are canceled. Not just for today and tomorrow, but until you fix your problem. Well, you have an appointment with destiny, the fulfillment of your unlimited potential. By starting to practice Hatha Yoga, you are fixing and maintaining the body properly, tuning up your Ferrari and getting it ready for the drive. Finally, you can really go somewhere.

Now we turn our attention from the car to the driver, the mind. The physical practice of yoga will help to condition the mind so it is a suitable partner for your newly purified and integrated body. Through Raja Yoga we will do for the mind what Hatha Yoga has done for the body. Only then can the marriage of these two suitable partners take place, allowing us to create a proper home for the Spirit, and invite it to join the body and the mind in their new temple.

Let me clear up something here. I said earlier that yoga was invented in order to still the body and prepare it for meditation. But some students misunderstand what that means. The reason we want the body and mind calm and relaxed is not just so we can sit on a cushion with our eyes closed; that's not the ultimate goal. Instead of the usual terminology of the "meditative state," think of it more as a *receptive state*, being *open* to the Spirit and inviting integration of the mind and the body. That is where we want to go. When you go to your first yoga class, your first real meditation will begin!

Without an intelligent and disciplined mind, you will recklessly drive your finely tuned-up car all over the road. Every day you are driving in Manhattan, on the gridlocked Avenue of the Americas during rush hour. You can't really open up the engine there, fire up all of your car's supernatural horsepower. You can't even get out of first gear! No, to really enjoy the $300,000 Ferrari or Lamborghini, you have to take it out on Highway 15 from California to Las Vegas, late at night, and then you can get it up to sixth gear, and really experience what you have under the hood. Nobody knows how much power they truly possess—how much heart power, physical power, mental power, spiritual power—until they can train their mind to a point at which they can silence all the unnecessary chatter and choose a real destination.

You will also require the will to *insist* on going—even when people are telling you you're stupid to do so—and the discipline to make yourself try over and over again, to never give up no matter what the obstacles, until you reach your goal. You need both mental toughness and physical toughness. In all there are five qualities of mind that you will have to instill: faith, self-control, determination, concentration and patience. Like the eight forms of yoga, they all operate interdependently and simultaneously. The good news is that you're already learning them. As you continue to improve your body in Bikram Yoga classes, you will also naturally increase all five Raja Yoga powers. And your mind will be tested and toughened under the duress that only my Torture Chamber and my unrelenting Dialogue can supply. You will become a distraction-proof, emotion-proof, mood-proof, attitude-proof yogi, because you have entered into cosmic consciousness. Here's how.

First, understand that the mind is at once the most important and the most complicated subject in human life. With a foundation of mental strength, you can truly accomplish anything.

Without control of mind, you can do nothing. You have something, but you don't know how to use it. The greatest challenge we face as human beings is controlling and properly using our own minds.

The mind is the communications system between the physical body and the Soul or Spirit; its primary responsibilities are to control the body and supply the Spirit with immediate and exact information. When the mind instead gives distracted and wrong information, the Spirit cannot govern properly—in fact, it cannot assume control at all. The ego-driven mind has had to rule for itself, and now it *does not want to* give up its ultimate authority over your life. This is a bitter, perverse fact about human beings, but it is the truth.

Without proper training, the mind will continue to give you the wrong information and divert your focus from your Spiritual goals. The way it does that so successfully is with fear and desire— its primary weapons. Like a drug dealer, the mind gets us addicted to these two opposite but conjoined emotions, and when we are constantly reacting to our attractions and aversions to people, things and situations, we can't see what really is and reopen the channels to our true Self, the Spirit. That's why I say that the mind has become our worst enemy.

To overcome this will not be easy. The weak mind is evergrowing, constantly feeding on your fears and negative habits. And as my guru taught me, the natural human attraction to something negative is *nine times* more powerful than our gravitational pull toward the positive—another very inconvenient fact.

In the philosophy of yoga we say there are five big negative behaviors, or Don'ts, which collectively are called *Yama* (in Sanskrit). They are: harming or injuring others; stealing; lying; possessiveness or greed; and neglecting or rejecting the Divine. The five Do's, or *Niyama*, are: keeping the body and mind pure; self-discipline; training the senses; studying the Divine; and surrendering to it. Now think of your own life: Why are you so often drawn to the *Yama*, things you know are bad for you? Why is it so hard to resist them, to get off your fat, lazy butt and go to yoga class? The power of negative attraction. Negative attitudes and emotions are like black holes in space, so powerful that they swallow everything that passes in front of their mouths, so even light cannot escape.

Resisting them demands much mental strength and supreme control. By regularly practicing Hatha Yoga and developing your faith, self-control, determination, concentration and patience, you can break those powerful distractions. This will then help you to perform your Karma Yoga and eventually attain mental peace. None of us is born with the perfect mixture of all five requisite mental qualities, just as we aren't born with strength, flexibility and balance in the body. But all five are within everyone's reach.

In the West, you always try to train your minds what to do, or *Niyama*. In India, we are trained what not to do first, the *Yama*. Either way, *you* must learn moderation and balance.

Faith

This may surprise you, as people often don't think of faith as a function of the mind. To illustrate why it belongs here—why it's absolutely vital to the control of the mind—let me tell you a little story.

The holiest man in India takes a journey through the Himalayas. At 85, he's also a billionaire, but he's renounced all that, giving his wealth and belongings to needy children. Today he's traveling barefoot through the snow, back to his guru's *ashram* to preach to the children and engage in Spiritual contemplation in the twilight of his life. Climbing up one of the higher peaks, his foot slips, and he starts to fall from a steep cliff into a deep chasm. As he falls, he cries out, "Oh, God! All my life I've tried to do everything for everybody else, sacrificing everything that I've earned through the sweat of my brow and the utter fulfillment of my Karma Yoga so that I may find a little peace at the end of my days and contemplate your mercy in solitude! How can you let me die this way, with my life as of yet unfulfilled?! How can this be your will?"

Suddenly, his body hits a small tree growing out from the side of the cliff, and he grabs on for dear life. Opening his eyes, he sees that he is suspended thousands of feet above broken rocks, with no way up and no way safely down. The little sapling is barely enough to support his weight, and he realizes that very soon either the tree will break or his grip will slip. So he prays to God: "Lord, in your infinite wisdom you have seen fit to dangle me above a most painful and untimely death. Everything I have done, I've done for you. Please help me—don't let me die in this way. I'll do anything you ask, anything at all—I promise to go back to work and build more temples. I'll feed the hungry. Anything, but please, please, please save me!"

God answers, "Yes, my son, why are you screaming!"

The holy man is filled with joy, and cries, "Oh, loving, kind, merciful God! I knew you would come to this poor beggar's aid! Please help me leave this place in safety, that I might continue to praise your glorious name!"

God tells him, "Just let go, and I will catch you, my son."

For a full five minutes, everything is completely quiet. Finally, the hanging holy man calls out, "Is there anybody *else* out there who can help me?"

For 85 years of his life, the holiest man in India says he believes in God. But when his faith is finally put to the test, he refuses to surrender his life to God out of fear of mortality. His life was almost over anyway; what did he have to lose? If he had truly given his life to God, then why couldn't he let go of the branch? The answer is simple: He lacked faith.

Faith is the essential ingredient in the practice of life, and supplies the foundation for controlling the mind. With faith, all things are possible—you just have to believe. In order to aspire to Self-Realization, you must first have faith in your Self, which at the end of the day is belief in God. Since Godliness is in all of us, how can you profess to believe in God if you don't believe in yourself? How can you ever realize anything in which you have no faith?

People who lack faith still go to temple, church or mosque, looking for answers. When they are physically sick, they go to a hospital; when they are mentally sick, they see a psychiatrist and fill a prescription for Prozac or some other pharmaceutical poison. I don't go to any of these places—why should I? I am not physically, mentally or spiritually sick, because I believe in my Self, I believe in you, and I believe in my subject: yoga. I *know* that because you are holding on to your foot, kicking your leg out and locking your knee for 60 seconds in my class today, that you will feel better tomorrow. Without true faith, belief doesn't mean anything, and the phrase "I believe in God" is just a bunch of empty words.

I learned to have faith in myself by first establishing faith in my guru. If he had ever told me to open the window and jump out, I would honestly have done it in the blink of an eye. I would never have hesitated, because that man had proven to me, time and time again, that his only concern was my success in life. Out of love, respect, loyalty and *faith*, I would never think twice about doing what my guru asked because I always believed in his love for me. This proved not just his worth to me, but *my worth*, you see? If he loved me the way he so clearly did, then I must have been lovable; I was worthy. From this, I got what you call self-esteem.

But you didn't have a guru, you tell me. You don't have the proof like mine, which would give you a bedrock belief in your own self-worth, which would give you true faith in the world outside you, in life itself. That's all right; no problem. To me, when I hear this, it's like you're saying, "I have a slipped disc" or, "I have a rotator cuff injury." You have a psychological injury and I have the prescription, Bikram's Rx, that I know will cure this mental problem just as it cures the physical ones.

I have faith in you. Already. And through my yoga I will transfer that faith to you, like Bishnu Ghosh did to me, and your own belief in yourself will grow inside you. I've seen it happen a million times. At the very foundation of my teachings, the way yoga was taught to me, is the knowledge that *there is nobody bad in this world*. We are all Gods and Goddesses. Through yoga you will see this and you will internalize that belief, as you learn to like yourself, love yourself and take care of yourself. To respect yourself. The purpose of my life is to make people realize the goodness buried in themselves—that they deserve to be happy, and they can be.

This happens in two very important ways, one that's very personal and internal and the other having to do with externals and other people. First, when you begin to honor your body by practicing Hatha Yoga, your relationship to that body changes. Now you have pride in it and begin to have faith in yourself. You can begin to let go of your bad habits: smoking, drinking too much, whatever. It takes five seconds, because when you do yoga you both love and like yourself. You know the value of your life. You realize that you can enjoy life better not drinking rather than drinking, or doing other things that defile your temple. Then you come to see yourself not as a slave to your bad habits, but as someone who has mastered them, and what do you get? More self-esteem—more than you can even imagine. In changing your bad habits and making choices that serve you instead of hurt you, you reestablish faith in your Self.

The second way yoga builds faith is through the community, the gathering of fellow souls in the class. Let's say somebody comes in who is not successful, and not very happy. Maybe she had a bad experience with a boyfriend, maybe she's even taking drugs. Or it can be someone else who is outwardly very successful—a lawyer or an engineer, he has a great job, a nice wife, cute little kids. But deep down he's not happy either; something is missing. The good news is, some friend of theirs bought them a yoga class as a present and finally one of them comes to the studio and what do they see? There are 50 people there and the other 49 are all smiling. So they can't help but think, Why not me?

Then they take the class and afterward their feet don't touch the ground. They fly through the air and they feel high without drugs or alcohol. They've never had that feeling in their life— maybe they're 30, 40, 50 years old, it doesn't matter—and now they can't wait to have that feeling again tomorrow. Everyone else in the class is nice to them, helps them, begins to influence them positively, so they see you *can* achieve your goals; you don't have to give up. We call this kind of community or influential group *satsang,* and it's a very powerful force. (A group that negatively influences its members is called *asatsang.*)

Other people's happiness and success rubs off on you. It's like when it's cold outside and your car doesn't start. That doesn't mean that you take the car and dump it in the junkyard, right? You just need a jump. All you have to do is go next door and ask, "Can you jump-start my car?" There's nothing wrong with you or your car; you just need a little help. And the belief the teacher and the other students in yoga class have in you jump-starts your own cold battery. They charge you with their faith, and then, after a while, you recognize your own faith, your own power.

Practicing Faith

When confronted with a choice in life get in the habit of asking yourself, Does this action (or nonaction) show faith in myself, the belief that I have godliness inside of me? Or does it demonstrate disrespect for myself, and suggest that my body and I really aren't that worthy? Your ego-mind doesn't want you to have this intelligent dialogue with yourself before you act. It wants to drive, to be in control, and for the rest of you to be unconscious in the backseat. And since negative pull is stronger than positive, it will often want to take you in the wrong direction.

But you know already, inside, what is right and what is wrong. When you bring these life choices out into the open and examine them, it becomes clear that the negative (*Yama*) choices make disrespectful statements about you. When you make conscious choices, it's easier for you to resist negativity and disrespecting yourself. As your belief in your Self grows with your practice, this becomes easier still, and asking yourself these questions before you act becomes a good habit, one you'll want to keep. It's so simple, really—trust me.

After you acquire true belief in yourself, you must develop the moral strength necessary to see it through, and to act on that belief—in other words, self-control.

Self-Control

This second element of a strong mind is also known as moral discipline. Self-control requires practice, and practice requires discipline. By controlling our minds, we acquire the mental strength necessary to make the distinction between *want* and *need*. This difference is even greater than the difference between good and bad, so huge and so crucial that these may be the two most important words in the English language—in any language. Life can be heaven or it can be hell; it all hangs on those two words. If you can judge and make a decision between what you want and what you need, then you can have the best life.

How do we make that distinction? Use your mind, your Raja Yoga logic. When your gas tank is empty, can you drive the car? No, you cannot. That means you need the gas. Technically, mechanically, you have no choice. Now, let's say you want to have a jumbo-size Mocha Frappuccino in your cup holder to make it a nice drive. Fine. But do you *need* that beverage to drive the car? No. It's a want, not a need.

First you need to fulfill your needs. Then you have choices; you can decide where you want to go. You want to go to Palm Springs? You want to go to the airport? Decide—it's up to you. But you can't go anywhere without the gas.

We want everything. Your mind tells you, "I want this, I want that, I want money, I want a house, I want happiness, I want sex, I want success, I want . . ." Again, it's trying to distract and confuse you, for you to equate wanting these things with needing them. But to want something is merely to crave, or desire, it. A need is a necessary duty or obligation.

It's okay to want. As we go through life, we may want to have a nice house, good food, fine clothes, and the best education. There is nothing wrong with desiring the best this life has to offer, but first things first. Before you attempt to satisfy your wants, you must be responsible in fulfilling your physical, mental, emotional, spiritual and financial needs. Being a slave to desire causes us to neglect our real needs. And in the culture of materialism, desire is rampant. Our downfall here comes when we expect that having things we want will satisfy us; that's what capitalism and materialism teach us. Thinking that way, when we feel the incredibly brief, transitory kind of satisfaction or happiness that getting a new toy brings, we confuse it with the real, deep, permanent satisfaction that is available to us. We lose our focus on reaching the state of joy that you get from practicing your Hatha, Raja and Karma Yoga.

Practicing Self-Control

The essential thing here is to distinguish between want and need and to keep those two things in their proper order. So again, you make the distinction explicit, bring it out into the open and defy your sneaky mind. When you feel yourself wanting something, don't beat yourself up for having desires. Just ask, Do I want this thing, or do I truly need it? Will it be a fun diversion, or will it really help me to get where I want to go?

You may conclude that it's just a want, then go ahead and get it, and that's fine. You may say, "Nah, it's just a superficial want; I don't need it. I'm going to concentrate on what's truly important and in ten minutes I'll have forgotten that I even wanted it."

Both answers are good answers; it's choosing *consciously* that matters. You will find, though, that labeling wants as such—having to admit to yourself that you don't really need them—takes so much of the power out of your cravings that you will start to consistently favor the needs. It's really the confused idea that we need something that makes us want it so badly. Plus, the slight delay, just the time it takes to ask and answer this question, takes a lot of the steam out of this heedless rush to have something. Want loses momentum, and the balance swings back toward taking care of business.

Developing self-control circles back to faith, the first quality of mind. If you lacked faith and did not believe in your Self, then there would be no motivation to achieve moral discipline. Faith allows you to do that, and self-control reinforces and rewards that faith. Then, the next quality to be instilled is willpower, or determination.

Determination

Your willpower must say "no" when no is required, overcoming fear and desire. When you feel angry, greedy, or naughty, you know it is wrong to act on such impulses, and you must rely on your willpower to prevail. When presented with a better but more difficult choice, your determination must lead you to say, "Yes, I will."

Here's one use of willpower that's extremely difficult to master: Responding with kindness to people who act out against you. And yet all the wise teachers from Jesus on down tell you that you must turn the other cheek. No matter how great the justification, if you react with anger and try to hurt the offender in return, things will only continue to worsen. If you walk away from a negative encounter peacefully, you are the winner. The person who tried to hurt you may even realize his or her mistake and eventually, they may learn from those mistakes and become a better human being.

Why is not responding to another person's anger so hard? Just as negative forces generally have more power than positive ones, another fact of life or human nature is that the right way is almost always the hard way. Life is a battlefield, and to win the battle and perform your Karma Yoga, you have to be the strongest soldier in the army. Plus, if you listen to the teachings of the great yogis, sages, masters and avatars of the world, you will hear the universally acclaimed truth that suffering is the only way to develop true compassion. Hell is the only way to get to heaven.

To continue choosing the hard way requires enormous determination. Earlier in this book I invoked Mahatma Gandhi and the slogan he gave to India's independence movement: "Do or die." In the spirit of Gandhi's great words, we must learn to be determined in our minds so that we can reclaim control of our lives. And we can do that through the vehicle of the body, using our Hatha Yoga to develop Raja Yoga.

While teaching my yoga class, I talk about the need for English bulldog determination in order to perform one's Karma Yoga. A bulldog's jaw has the ability to lock, maintaining an unshakable grip that can be released only through choice or physical death. This is true willpower. And it is in the furnace of my Torture Chamber that this quality is forged. You're in there holding an *asana*, shaking and shuddering, your every muscle crying out, and your mind is yelling at you to quit, to please bring an end to this mental and physical pain. That's when I come to your rescue by sweetly telling you, *"Just try to kill yourself, honey."*

Does this mean that I want to see my students physically die in my yoga class? Absolutely not; that disturbs the rest of the class, makes a mess on the carpet, and is very difficult to explain to their families. (Plus, if they expire, how will they ever pay for their next 10 lessons?) When I say *kill yourself*, I'm talking about killing your false, lowercase self and overcoming the slavery of your own mind. Raised by parents who tell them, "Take it easy, honey—just do the best that you can" and, "Don't hurt yourself, honey," people get brainwashed to expect very little of themselves. I say, break free of the bonds that have held you back from achieving your true potential in life.

You'll see then that Hatha Yoga is not just about the postures, and that technique is not all you are learning. Equally important is the determination we learn in order to perform the postures. Trying the right way, giving 100 percent sincere effort, gives you 100 percent of the benefit, even if you can only do a posture 1 percent correctly! Never give up. Never slack off. It is only through disciplined willpower that physical health, mental peace and Self-Realization can be achieved.

Practicing Determination

Obviously, practicing in a Bikram Yoga school is like going to the determination factory and buying mass quantities of willpower at wholesale prices. However, it's also true that the specific challenge you choose to build willpower with really doesn't matter; it's the trying itself that counts. The task just needs to be sufficiently challenging or daunting to require willpower, and like yoga, to offer attractive enough rewards to make the effort seem worthwhile.

So set an additional goal for yourself outside the studio, something that would be very hard for you to attain, but that would be oh-so-satisfying. Now *double it*. That's right. Not climbing Mount Everest, but climbing Mount Everest on one leg! Not earning a million dollars to give to charity, but making and giving away 2 million dollars! Remember, we are only limited by our imaginations, our thoughts and dreams. Everything is attainable with enough hard work, once you understand your true destination.

Concentration

I've told you that in India our custom has been to place the education of our children in the hands of gurus. And in our religious mythology the gods and goddesses did the same thing. One great sage who had been chosen to teach the gods' sons to become warriors was the enlightened teacher named Dronacharya. One day, Dronacharya assembled all the boys together for a test. He lined them up side by side in a great field, with nothing on the horizon but a lone tree standing miles in the distance, holding in its branches a wooden bird. Equipped with a stout bow and a single arrow each, the boys stood at attention, awaiting the command of their teacher.

He told them, "Everyone aim at the bird. Then, when I call your name, shoot at the bird."

Approaching the first boy on the line, Dronacharya asked him, "What do you see at the end of the field, young warrior?"

"I see the bird, Sir!" the boy answered bravely.

"What else do you see?" inquired the Master.

"I see the tree, Sir!"

"What else do you see?"

"I see the sky and everything else behind the tree, Sir!"

"*Wrong!*" Dronacharya roared. "Next boy!"

The same questions were repeated to 99 more boys, and after successfully identifying the bird in the tree, they gave 99 different answers to the next question, all of which received a thundering "Wrong! Next boy!" from their teacher. From the dew on the leaves, to the sap on the trunk, to the sun in the sky, to the wind in the branches, no reply would satisfy Dronacharya.

Finally, he came to Arjun, his favorite student and the most promising young warrior of all. (I told you about him before; he will become the warrior whose dialogue with Lord Krishna on the eve of a great battle forms the epic story that defines Karma Yoga.) The last boy in the line, Arjun stood unmoving, and stared unblinking into the sun, which was starting to set behind the lone tree.

"What do you see, Arjun?" his guru demanded.

"I see the bird, Sir!" he smartly replied.

"What else can you see?"

"Just the bird, Sir!" Arjun answered.

"What part of the bird?"

"I see the head of the bird, Sir!"

"What part of the head?"

"I see the left eyeball, Sir!"

"What *else* do you see?"

"Nothing, Sir!"

"*Shoot!*" the guru commanded.

Arjun released his arrow and pierced the left eye of the bird, passing the test.

The fourth element of a strong mind, as illustrated by this story, is the power of *concentration*. When you concentrate, all good things in the world are yours. Let's say you have a son who is failing in school, can't get his work done on time and flunks his tests, while your daughter is smart, clever and a straight-A student. They're both very intelligent; the only difference between them is their ability to concentrate.

You must also be able to focus. You must have an *aim* in life, and you cannot blink your eyes or take your eyes off of the target. If you do, you are scattered, thinking of five things at once, like the other young warriors. You can't keep your mind on any one thing for 10 seconds. Then you are *aimless*, with no real goal in life and no hope of reaching Self-Realization. And having too many choices keeps you from being able to concentrate and get things done. In India students must declare in the eighth grade what course of study they will pursue, whether it's the arts, science or commerce. But the student doesn't make that decision, his or her teacher and guru decide, and *that's it*! Not like here, where people go to four kinds of graduate schools until they're 40 and still don't know what they want to be when they grow up.

With concentration, you will finally be capable of making a commitment, maintaining your aim and your purpose and doing your job, no matter how long it takes. I like to say that concentration brings life to your life. This power is what meditation was invented to develop; it trains you to focus completely on one thing and one thing only, beginning with a mantra or the breath. And as I've explained, my yoga class does the same thing, driving all thoughts from your mind except what you need to concentrate on to successfully perform each posture. You have to—you have no choice!

Do you know how hard it is to concentrate for 10 seconds while attempting one yoga posture? Imagine that you are listening to me lead you through *Utkatasana*, the Awkward posture. You're having some difficulty balancing as you stretch out your arms in front of you, trying to sit deeper in an imaginary chair, keeping your wrists, feet and knees 6 inches apart, heels directly behind the toes, chest up, weight in the heels, leaning back as if you are trying to fall down backward, way back, farther back—now change!

In only 10 seconds, it's over. Could you have possibly thought about anything else during those 10 seconds without falling back on your butt? Besides the physical demands, the words of the Dialogue take command of your mind. In 10 seconds I give you 20 things to remember. I'm screaming while you're desperately, continuously and simultaneously communicating between your body, my words and your mind. That's concentration power, my friend. And when you have it, no one can steal your peace.

Practicing Concentration

To do a diagnostic test on your ability to concentrate, try a quick meditation right now. Sit comfortably, either in a chair with your feet flat on the floor and your spine straight against the back of the chair, or on the floor with your legs crossed, spine straight. Close your eyes and think to yourself, "God, God, God, God . . ." Or choose a temporary mantra for yourself, any little word that comes to mind, and repeat that silently, over and over. Within about five seconds, I bet you'll be thinking "Sex, sex, sex . . . money, money, money . . . food, food, food . . ." You'll open your eyes and wonder why you were sitting there, and what the hell it was that you were supposed to be doing. You can almost hear your mind laughing at you.

Do not be alarmed; this is completely normal. You need more concentration power. To develop it, you may want to learn some meditation techniques and do them regularly in addition to your

Hatha Yoga practice. In any case, training the mind to concentrate takes time: When you catch a wild lion in the jungle, it may take awhile before it's ready to perform in the circus. Time is essential to developing every part of mind control, and this prolonged and pointed pursuit brings up the last mental quality you will need, which is patience.

Patience

Suppose you have developed faith, self-control, determination and concentration, but you still don't have the mental peace you seek. Why? You are lacking the fifth quality of mind. Your journey to Self-Realization will be a long one; it's not an overnight thing, like they FedEx it to you or something. This is a lifelong process you've just started; you are going to need patience.

Imagine that you are driving cross-country from Los Angeles to New York. You've spent weeks planning your trip, mapping out the best possible route, deciding which cities and towns to stay in and which sights to see. You've made reservations at five-star, trendy hotels and had your mechanic rotate the tires, change the oil and perform a tune-up on your trusty vehicle. You've packed your car with food and CDs, and called all your friends along the way to let them know when you'll be passing through. Finally, the big day arrives, and you get in your car, top off the tank, and hit the road. You get as far as Phoenix, and suddenly you say to yourself, "My God, this is taking too long! Forget it!" So you make a quick U-turn and head back to L.A., tires screeching. What happened? Before you left you understood intellectually that the entire trip would cover over 3,500 miles and that it would take at least six days, but you only made it through half a day. When faced with the reality of it, you ran out of patience.

It is said that patience is a virtue. Too bad nobody possesses any. I have developed some patience through all of the obstacles I have overcome in my life—but I still don't like using it. Time is the only thing I fear in this life, and I refuse to waste my precious time by waiting for tomorrow, next week, next year or the next life to do anything. Who knows what could happen? Driving home from teaching class tonight, I could crash my car and end my life; tomorrow may never come. There is so much left for me to experience in my life, and so much work to be done that I haven't got time to wait. Remember, I told you before: Performing your Karma Yoga and doing your job on Earth means not just doing it honestly and properly but doing it on time.

However, when it comes to my students and yoga, I always do my best to be patient. Many students who come to class will be practicing for the rest of their lives, and not everyone's progress is exceptionally fast. It's like my guru used to say: You can't beat a donkey into a horse. How effective would I be as a yoga teacher if I lacked the patience to let my students struggle through their own difficulties, even if they don't listen to me as well as they should? Should I kick them out? "Sorry, honey. You've been coming for over six months now, and you still can't lock the goddamn knee. Go home." No. As the teacher, I must have the necessary patience to guide them so that they can heal themselves.

Practicing Patience

One very simple but effective way to practice patience is by using *Savasana*, something you already know how to do from my class. I told you before that despite its apparent simplicity, for many, many students, this is the most difficult posture of all. How could that be, since it only involves lying there still, like a corpse? The real challenge is not physical but mental. The devious, disobedient mind doesn't want you to clear away all the useless thoughts it's throwing at you; hear the calm voice of sanity beyond the chatter of thoughts, and that's a threat to the mind's rule over your life. So when you stop your activity and simply lie there and attempt to be calm and relaxed, it will redouble its noisy attack. The mind will throw everything it's got at you to make you scratch your nose, wipe your face, scratch your ass, get up and go to the bathroom or get a drink of water. Anything to break your intention.

That's what makes *Savasana* a great patience-builder. All you need to do—not that it's easy, by any means—is wait the mind out, exercise patience; in the end you will win. In class we can use *Savasana* only in very short spurts, usually for 20 seconds. When you're at home, and you can spare five minutes to help save your life, just lie down wherever you are, in whatever clothes you are wearing, and rest in *Savasana* for five minutes.

Find a spot on the ceiling to focus on. Remember, the eyes are open the whole time. You're flat on your back, legs straight, heels together, arms by your sides, completely relaxed. Palms face up toward the ceiling. Concentrate on your breath, inhaling deeply and then exhaling fully (through the nose at all times). All you need to do is wait for the chatter to die down and the five minutes to be up. Doing this exercise daily will not only increase your patience but will also calm and prepare you mentally and physically for the rest of your day's activities.

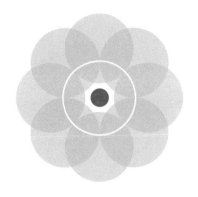

CHAPTER ELEVEN

The Four Stages of Life: A Road Map to Happiness

NOW YOU ARE REALLY GETTING SOMEWHERE. YOU'VE BEGUN to claim your birthright by maintaining a healthy body and cultivating a peaceful mind. Now you can begin to invite your true Self into the magnificent castle you're creating, or to put it another way, to open communication between your body and mind and the Spirit that lies buried within you. As you will see, the energy and power of that Spirit is infinite, and now you have access to that force. As my guru said: *"Yoga brings out the hidden forces of the latent power to make you into your real self."*

But that doesn't mean your work is done and that you can just wait passively for the power of enlightenment to pour over you. You must actively carry out a new life plan. It's about slowly, carefully planting, cultivating and eventually harvesting the divine. Thinking life through before you live it is part of Vedanta Yoga: the way of philosophy, thoughts and ideas. Or, to go back to my favorite analogy of all-time—cars, what else?—you have to have a map to show you the way to that destination. *How*, by what routes, will you get to supreme happiness? And you will need signs along the way, checkpoints and mileage markers by which to measure your progress. Are you far enough along to arrive in time, while you're still alive? You can't keep track of how you are doing by the things you possess, such as your clothes, your job, your car or a diploma. This is life progress we are talking about, Spiritual progress.

The map of life I am offering you comes from the ancient wisdom of India and the yogic tradition. Again, I don't hold up India as a model because we are all so perfect, but because I believe this life plan can be valuable to all. Because this is America, and we no longer live in ancient times but in modern ones, this framework will need some modifications for your use. In fact, because you live here in 21st-century America, you have advantages and opportunities that the ancients didn't have and that Indians today still don't possess. Take what works for you from the traditional plan, then customize it for your personal circumstances and preferences. Take the best from both worlds. Again, what's right is what works.

Remember also that this ancient four-stage plan was always an ideal; not everyone can pull it all off, and that's okay, too. But overall it's the best way I know to systematically approach your life, carrying your yoga with you as the master key.

In yoga we see life as sectioned into four sequential stages, of varying lengths, which when fulfilled are the foundation for Self-Realization. The first part is called *Brahmacharya* (which translates literally as "renunciation" or "celibacy"), the second one *Garahasthya* (family life), the third part *Banaprasthya* (nonattachment), and the fourth and last one is called *Sannyas* (asceticism). Each of these four parts is necessary for fulfilling the promise of the whole. Enlightenment is reached step by step by step. You never start from the middle and you can't finish in the middle. This also has the advantage of allowing us—and now you—to divide the daunting process of living into smaller and more manageable pieces.

To complete this journey you will need all of your bodily strength and willpower, all of the newfound qualities you are instilling through your practice. Why? For one thing, people usually don't want to go on to the next stages of life. Whether it is moving from the first quarter, childhood, into the second, adulthood, or from the second to the third, each change is marked by fear. People want to remain in the lower level because they think they're going to miss something, or it's going to be too hard to move on. Middle-aged people miss their college life; they don't want to grow up. But you have to live appropriately, in a way that suits the stage you are in. You can't have one foot in high school and one foot in raising a family. We say: "You can't have two feet in two boats." You know why? Because if you divide yourself and stand in two floating, moving boats, your ass ends up in the water!

People are afraid to let go because they don't know the rewards of moving forward, the joy of a higher level of consciousness. Remember the dying billionaire clinging to the tree? He was afraid to let go and miss a single day of life, even though God was personally reassuring him that he would be moving on to a higher level—he didn't want to give anything up, even to gain so much more. That's because he was not a true yogi.

With the help of a disciplined yoga practice you can understand yourself, where you came from, where you are today, where you should be tomorrow, and where you'll end up the day after tomorrow. You are educated in life, not just living one. With this yogic instruction to follow you can get a PhD in life, summa cum laude.

First Stage: Building the Foundation

The first part of life, *Brahmacharya*, begins at birth and lasts until you finish your education. In it you need to learn who you are, why you came to this Earth—your duty, your path—how you will achieve your duty, and what kind of tools you will need along the way. This is your foundation. The foundation of my life and my personality is like the Empire State Building's. Nobody in this world can convince me to do anything against my heart or my mind because my country, my guru, my parents, and my friends set it in the right place, the right way. You can change a window or you can change a brick, but you cannot shake that foundation.

Whether from the East or the West, children universally are incapable of making responsible life choices on their own. This problem is sometimes compounded because parents are often too emotionally bound to their children to properly discipline them or show them the right way to live. You wouldn't have a heart surgeon operate on his own daughter, would you, cracking open her chest and cutting into the tiny heart he loves so much? He might lose his nerve because he wouldn't be objective—he's too close, too emotionally attached. Even when a situation is not life-or-death, parents can be their children's worst enemies. They're so afraid something will happen to them, they say, "No, don't try that, you might get hurt!" "Don't eat that, you might get an upset stomach!" Through the desire to keep their children from suffering, parents can make kids very weak. Sometimes parents who truly want happiness and fulfillment for their children have to simply get out of the way.

That's why for so many generations Indians lived the *Brahmacharya* stage under the guidance of a guru, who takes over where the parents leave off. In fact, this was the law: As soon as your son turned six or seven years old, he had to be sent to a guru's *ashram*. *Ashrams* were for boys only; girls were sent to convent schools, which provided similar discipline and a solid foundation. Young men and women were kept far apart, which helps to maintain *Brahmacharya*, celibacy. Proximity to the opposite sex is just too distracting. Even if a boy's mother wanted to come and visit him, she had to be met outside of the school grounds. (Strong attachments to one's father and brothers were discouraged also—you should be focused on your guru and his teachings—but they were at least allowed to visit.) Even Mrs. Indira Gandhi was never allowed inside an *ashram*, until a special arrangement was made.

When you're young, the guru is like a sculptor and you are the clay. Clay could be made into anything—a statue of Jesus Christ or a statue of Hitler, you follow me? The clay will do nothing by itself, and only responds to the hands that shape it. Depending on the quality of the clay, and the ability of the artist, you and the guru can create yourself as a lawyer, an engineer, a doctor, a singer, a wise man, a philosopher, a yoga teacher, you name it. A real master can see what good qualities a young person has: What is his potential? Where does her destiny lie? Bishnu Ghosh could look at a kid like me with his piercing black eyes and see in one second who that kid was destined to become. Didn't matter if it was a poor kid begging for money on the street or one from a wealthy background; he could see inside them both and he'd help them both.

The Spiritual master, or *sensei*, as the Japanese would call him, enforces strict rules and regulations, balancing out destructive natures and allowing children to clear away the obstructions of early adulthood. A guru will teach lessons that last a lifetime. Because of this, a guru traditionally comes before mother, before father, even before God, in my country. The guru-disciple relationship is the most important relationship in human life! Now I know parents in this country don't want to hear *that*, but bear with me.

Child-rearing was done this way because it works. The hard way, the right way. This is a delicate, tricky and even irresponsible stage of life for most children, right through adolescence, and requires special caution and care. Children aren't bad; they're simply not ready to operate safely on their own. Sure, every kid wants to get out of the house and get a job far away, or maybe go to school at a college or university across the country. And here in the West we think that's good, saying, "Go, stand on your own two feet." But what do they do on those feet? Are they happy to move far away so they can have sex more often, acquire drugs more readily, and ignore their responsibility toward their family? Even before they leave home, junior-high and high-school kids today are getting into all kinds of trouble—and picking up all kinds of mental and physical diseases.

All I know is that at the *ashram* there was no time for smoking, drinking and fooling around. My guru beat me like a piece of raw steel beneath the blacksmith's hammer, making me bullet-proof, nailproof, fireproof, emotion-proof, everything-proof. He did this so that once he sent me out into the world, nobody could ever make a scratch on my body, my mind or my Spirit. I'm the most fortunate man in the world because I met him at an early age, and because of that, I am who I am today.

Another big difference between the way I was raised, in the guru system, and today's practice is that now we think that kids go to school to learn facts, that it's about getting them into pres-tigious schools like Harvard or Stanford, to get them high-paying jobs they don't even like. But Indian boys went to the *ashram* to learn everything about life, about the world and about Spiritual-ity. It was as much about ethics, as you would call it here, as it was about reading or math. That's missing here, and to me that's a big problem. To prepare our children to shape the future of our world, and for them to be happy, moral and productive adults, we must begin to cultivate ethics in them when they're very young. If you don't plant the right seed, you won't get the right fruit.

Say you put a little seed in the ground, you water it and nur-ture it, and then you wait for the seed to become a mighty tree. You sit beneath it, waiting patiently for the first beautiful fruit. Then one day you see a green lemon hanging in what you be-lieved to be your apple tree. You can't believe it; this is not what you wanted at all! So you get angry and scream at the tree. "I raised you all my life to be a beautiful apple tree, that I might have shade and fruit in my last years. I hate lemons!" Now, think about it: Who is to blame for the lemon, you or the tree? An ap-ple tree when properly nourished, will always provide sweet ap-ples. A lemon tree will always provide lemons. The truth is in the seed. Always.

First Stage: Here and Now

Okay, now you're depressed. I just explained to you how the way you were raised is no good and the way you are educating your children is all wrong. It's a hopeless situation. Not so! Gurus and *ashrams* are the traditional way, and for me they were the perfect way, but there are other ways. Look, even in India there are not many *ashrams* left. (There should be, but there aren't.) You didn't have a guru, nobody gave you the guidance and the discipline you needed? That's okay! Remember the most vital teaching from my guru: *"It's never too late, it's never too bad, and you're never too old or too sick to start from scratch once again."*

When you start to practice Hatha Yoga as an adult, you are born again. You start over; instantly, you get another chance. I give you a new life! Where is your guru? Understand that a guru does not necessarily have to be an Indian spiritual master. Anyone who offers you a good example of how to live your life could be considered a guru. Your parents might be good examples, or you may seek assistance elsewhere. Plus, many of you in the West choose to make important decisions primarily by yourself, independently, and that is a perfectly valid path. Just accept the expert guidance of those you admire; discover their methods and habits, and adopt them as your own. Think for yourself, but be sure to find something useful and beneficial to think about.

Here's the most incredible part: As you improve yourself through the practice of yoga, you can actually *become your own guru.* For you it will happen in the second quarter of life, not the first as in the traditional way. So what? This is how you will begin to know and to love yourself the way a guru would have. Yoga gives you an introduction to yourself, the person you never really knew, and you know what? I bet you will be pleased to meet you.

In my yoga classes and schools, you are presented with a cosmic mirror, in which you not only see yourself more clearly, but you can also see me, and through me, my guru, and through him, Paramahansa Yogananda, to all the great spiritual teachers and sages that have come before and passed down their wisdom through the ages. Together we will find your way, only now you will lead. I will tell you more about this in the next section, on the Second Stage, because that is where you will discover your Karma Yoga, taking on the guru's sacred duty.

"What about our kids?" you are asking. How can you raise them the right way in today's United States, where there are no *ashrams* and no traditional gurus? This is one of the most important questions we face in this country—and this time, my friend, the answer lies with you, not me.

When you practice yoga, you naturally—automatically—become more patient, which is like precious gold when it comes to parenting. And since you are less stressed and more relaxed, you will no longer be transmitting all that tension directly to your children. They feel it, believe me. Most important, through your practice you will be setting a better example.

You know that children always follow older people; they mirror them and kids imitate everything they see their parents do. Parents already know this, but sometimes they just can't control their own behavior, much less their kids', and that's when they set a bad example. How often have you seen a family in the car, the father driving, and then someone honks at him and then he rolls down the window and curses that other driver out? You know that as soon as those children get home, they will start calling each other those same nasty names. And they've learned at the same time that it's okay to show anger freely, that even their supposed role models can't control their emotions. Come on, parents, you can do better than that—and through yoga, you will.

When I grew up in India I never heard the word "stupid" or "idiot" come out of my father's mouth, and I never heard one curse word from either of my parents. Not one time. (I never used bad words myself until I came here, to Hollywood, where I heard them constantly.) Sure, my father and mother would argue or fight sometimes. But when they saw that we children were listening, they knew how to put the brakes on; they'd stop. From what I've seen, in many other families parents who are arguing can't stop themselves, no matter who's listening, until they think of the last, worst thing they can say to the other person—and then they say it. They can't disagree without taking it all the way. Through yoga you not only learn self-control, discipline, and patience, you also learn moderation. You don't have to take everything all the way anymore.

So you must set the right example, *showing* your kids the right way instead of just telling them what to do all the time. You get better results that way, and by showing instead of telling them "Do this; don't do that," you can also use their natural curiosity to guide them. My guru told me that when he was a young boy, his father would get up every morning and do 25 push-ups. And, naturally, the son would watch. This went on for a long, long time and then finally one morning my guru said to his father: "What are you doing? Every day you do these 25 push-ups, never less, never more. Why? What is this?"

"What have I been doing?" my guru's father replied. "I've been waiting for you to ask me about this." Then he explained the exercise and how it keeps you strong. "Thank God you finally asked me," the father continued, "because now I don't have to do them anymore. Starting tomorrow, *you* have to do them." So my guru did, and as I've said, he went on to become one of the greatest athletes of all time. And it was his curiosity, and a wise parent, that led him to it.

You will help your children's development enormously by taking them to a certified Bikram Yoga School and getting them to practice, starting as early as eight years old. There they will see adults showing respect for the teacher and each other. That's why my wife Rajashree's mother always took her to yoga school in India; she knew they were strict there. Over time, children will learn to act with respect for their elders and also to control their behavior—without their parents constantly having to be the disciplinarians. Some of my students have been coming here 35 years, and often they've brought their children along. Let me tell you, these kids, who are growing up 100 percent the American way in every other respect, are incredibly well-disciplined.

Kids who practice yoga learn to control their bodies and their breathing, and eventually gain better control over their minds and their emotions. These are incredibly important skills for young people—and very difficult to acquire. Nothing teaches them like yoga. Once children have these qualities, they can perform so much better at anything they choose, including academics.

Of course yoga will also help young people excel in sports, but I feel there's too much emphasis on athletics here in the United States. It seems that we take our kids for soccer, or swimming, so they can learn to compete and to win—and best of all, get a college scholarship! But even if your kid becomes a world champion, that doesn't mean he knows how to behave or that he will be happy. From what I've seen, such children are just as likely to develop a star athlete's attitude, to think they're a great person just because they're a great athlete, and to think only of themselves. In India we don't bring home Olympic gold medals—and we have more than one billion people. But we know how to treat people with civility, and kids there know how to behave and co-operate.

My son Anurag is 14 now, and Laju, our daughter, 16. I see how busy and pressed for time they are, and it's kind of crazy. Between after-school sports and all the other kinds of teams and clubs—plus all the homework they're given these days, my God!—children here don't really have time to practice yoga even if they want to. To me, the solution, and the way to implement the best of the traditional Indian way of child-rearing in America right now, is by offering yoga in all our schools. Maybe "offer" is the wrong word, since I think it should be mandatory, for all kids. I cannot overemphasize this and indeed I will return to it later when we talk about community service in the Third Stage of life.

When a baby is born, you have him or her inoculated against diseases. What we need to do is vaccinate all our children in the schools, public and private, with yoga instruction. Just one half-hour a day; that's all it would take to protect them for the rest of their lives. And what would it cost? Practically nothing. A few bucks for the teacher, maybe, though the schools could probably find volunteers. When you go before your school board and you propose yoga for the kids every day, they will ask you, who is going to teach them? And you just might find yourself answering, "I will." You'll be scared afterward—"What did I say?" But with your new yoga power and determination, you will figure it out and get it done. It will be so easy, you won't believe it, and you will be performing your Karma Yoga.

Some of my teachers are doing this already and so are a few schools around the country. Usually they are schools with no money, which serve poorer populations, because there, it seems, where we think there's nothing to lose, we are willing to take a chance. In the Namaste School in Chicago the 4- and 5-year olds (who are 90 percent black and Hispanic) start the day with *pranayama*, and they do more breath-work and postures throughout the day, including in PE. What better kind of physical education could there be? Again, yoga helps kids get their young bodies and minds more under control, so that they can learn. Just yelling at them, or sending them to stand in the corner, in a time-out, teaches them nothing. It just punishes, and creates anger and resentment, not love and mutual respect.

Right here in L.A. there's The Accelerated School, a K–8 inner-city charter school where yoga is a compulsory subject. The state of California tested their kids and found that they were physically fitter than the average for the school district; they also had fewer discipline problems and better grades. Of course the school gets great results! You don't have to test for me to know that those kids are going to succeed. The question is: Why doesn't every kid have the same advantage? Why only the so-called disadvantaged kids? Something is very screwed up, you must agree. Putting yoga in all the schools would be the most powerful force for good, to give all our children the proper First Stage of life, giving them the mortar and brick to build a solid foundation.

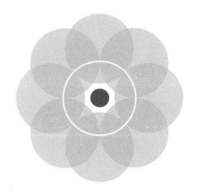

CHAPTER TWELVE

Second Stage, Part One: Love and Marriage

A wife loves her husband not for his own sake, dear, but because the Self lives in him. A husband loves his wife not for her own sake, dear, but because the Self lives in her.
— *The Upanishads (ancient Hindu scriptures)*

THIS SECOND QUARTER OF LIFE, GARAHASTHYA, IS THE LONgest one; it begins when you finish your education and lasts up until what we would call the retirement years. During this phase you find a job in your chosen area of expertise, then you get married and have children. (*Garahasthya* translates as "family life.")

249

You take care of your mother and father; your grandmother and grandfather, too. The other vitally important component in this stage is discovering and performing your Karma Yoga. That's a lot to deal with. So I'll describe each part separately, family first.

Family life and marriage is essentially about love. What is love? We are born to give and to try to understand the definition; this brings us closer to God. First you must learn how to like yourself, and then you begin to love your Self, the God within you. If we are wise we discover that we are love and God is love. Then we can make a true connection, a union between two minds, two bodies and two Spirits, whether with a parent, child, a neighbor, a friend, or a partner.

One example of pure love is mother love. Here's another story we tell in India, which demonstrates this concept.

> Once upon a time, in Calcutta, a boy fell deeply in love with a girl. But he waited. He finished college, he got a job and he said, "Okay, now I can take care of you. Let's get married."
>
> The girl said, "No. I cannot marry you, because you live with your mother and she controls you. I don't want to live with a mother-in-law who is always going to control me. I will always have fights with her. I don't want to marry you."
>
> "Okay," said the boy. "I will talk to my mother." So he does, and he comes back to the girl the next day and tells her, "Okay, I can live separately in an apartment with you and she won't disturb us."
>
> "No, no," says the girl. "She will come. Every mother controls her son in India."

"Okay, then we will move to another state," the boy offers.

"No," the girl replies, "she will come."

Exasperated, the boy asks, "What do you want me to do?"

The girl thinks a moment, then replies, "I will make you a deal. If you kill your mother, then I will marry you. And to prove it, you have to bring me her heart on a plate."

"How can you be so cruel and heartless?" the boy exclaims. Later, he goes to see his mother. He is clearly very sad, and his mother asks, "Son, what happened to you? Tell me."

So the boy tells his mother the whole story. The mother laughs. "That's all? Why didn't you tell me before? Your happiness is my happiness. Your life is my life. I'll do anything for you. Because I love you, happily I will die. I will lie down and you can cut my heart out. Here's the knife; now get to work!"

Together, the mother and son do this thing. The boy takes the still-warm heart and runs as fast as he can back to his girlfriend. Just as he is almost to her door, he slips and falls. The heart flies in the air, but he manages to catch it with the plate. He looks down at his mother's heart and it says to him, "Son, are you okay? Did you hurt yourself?"

That's mother love, real love. If you are a mother, you bring another Spirit onto this earth and you have a duty to that creation. A good mother will sacrifice anything for her children.

Much of the time, though, we are far from love. Instead, we project our fears and insecurities onto others. Then what should be a joyous and fulfilling part of life, a loving marriage, often becomes a source of pain, especially when people have not been raised with the proper foundation. Why do people fight and divorce? Lack of true, soul-to-soul communication. A man and a woman can speak to each other, but they are only moving their lips if there is no God, no mind and no Spirit in their words. "I love you, honey." "I miss you." It is not a question of saying these things, it is a question of feeling them, understanding them, *believing* them.

Most Americans seem to view divorce as a fact of life, an inescapable reality of adulthood. Marriages self-destruct or cannot be formed in the first place because, without yoga, neither party knows how to do it. It's like me owning the longest swimming pool in Beverly Hills—which I do—but not being able to go near it because I can't swim.

How then should we make and maintain the marriage commitment? Here is the most important requirement: To be successfully married to another, first you *must* create a marriage between your own body, mind and Spirit. In other words, you must practice yoga. That's how you improve yourself and become a worthy partner, and only then are you qualified to have a happy marriage.

As a 100 percent complete human being, you can now offer yourself to another unified body, mind, and Spirit who has achieved the same wholeness, the same humanity. You open your loving heart with the help of your intelligent mind. The moment you open it, you allow other hearts to connect with yours. If another person has a complete marriage like yours with their own body, mind and Spirit, then they will be able to see you as who you truly are. This quality is what draws *whole people* together.

In Western culture, men and women are too often shopping for partners; browsing, and looking at each other with a lot of expectations, but with very little investment. If they end up not liking the product they bought, they'll take it back, or throw it out and look for a replacement. That doesn't work.

In India, marriage is a very different kind of shopping—it's like buying a used car at auction. On the window there is a sign that reads, "As is." I cannot buy the car, then get home and open the hood and complain that there is no engine. Maybe the brakes aren't working. Now it's your car; you own it and you can't get your money back. You have to adjust and learn to live with it. Don't get me wrong; this isn't a foolproof method, and it's not one that many Americans are likely to adopt. But the principles behind it are true and universal. Let me show you what I mean by telling you my experience of marriage.

I've been very fortunate. When the time came, I let my parents decide whom I should marry; they knew better than I did what was best for me. My parents, along with my guru's son, Bisu, chose Rajashree to be my wife. She is a yogini and also dedicated to spreading the wisdom of yoga. She is the best partner for my life, and we've been married now for 22 years. Here's what I've come to understand from observing my parents and from my time with Rajashree: *Life is not about getting; life is about giving.* In India we say that if you try to get, in the end you lose, but if you try to give, in the end you win. Giving is the very essence, the purpose and the definition of marriage. You offer yourself unconditionally, not because you expect anything in return. Give, and have zero expectations.

Giving comes naturally to yogis because our way of life teaches us to give, to serve others, in order to perform our Karma Yoga. Remember the mantra my guru gave me? *"Serve your Self; you are born to give, not to get."*

The other crucial component of a successful marriage, one that's so often missing, is acceptance. If men and women don't try to "trade in" their mates at the first sign of problems, often they try instead to change that person, to make them become someone else they think they want. But real, pure love does not include the desire to change each other; it's about loving a person the way they are. Neither Rajashree nor I is perfect, that's for sure. But we do not criticize or expect to change each other, nor will we ever forsake each other. Again, yoga is what allows this to happen and true love to flourish: Once you two have learned to love and accept yourselves through yoga, you can more easily accept each other. You are focused on improving yourselves, not each other.

Yoga practice also teaches us how to make a long-term commitment. When we first meet our mate, that person seems to be the most beautiful, fascinating person on the Earth. But over time, we begin to take them for granted. If our life's destination is good sex and lots of fun for now, then the marriage is doomed to fail. But in our yoga practice we have come to embrace a lifelong journey, and we've learned the patience and determination to stay the course through all the highs and lows.

We know the rewards will be there if we only stick with it. So we are capable of seeing marriage in the same way—we know that the real destination is a lifetime of companionship and the gift of knowing someone as well as yourself, and we have a better chance of success. Remember, the best English translation for the word *yoga* is "marriage," or "union." And the best tool or guide for marriage is yoga as well.

Since I've been in this country I've actually arranged marriages myself, and I'm very good at it. I can tell whether or not people should be together. I have a student named Gary, who is also my friend. One day in class I told him, "Hey, Gary, I think you should marry Robin here." Robin is the daughter of two of my students, and she was right in front of me in the classroom. I've known her since she was a tiny girl. "You two go out," I told them. "No coochie-coochie, no touchy-touchy, and you see if I'm wrong." Well, they took my advice, and they got married the next week, without dating and before making love. Five hundred people were at the wedding, and when it was time for the first dance, Robin said to Gary, "I want to dance with my guru first, because he told me to marry you." They have been happily married for more than 15 years and have two beautiful children.

This ability to see who's compatible and who isn't, which I inherited from my guru, can get me in trouble. Once when another of my students was planning to marry I said, "Hey, don't do it. It's not going to last." And my student said, "Why not? We love each other *soooo* much." Yeah, whatever. I knew. So after three dramatic months they got divorced, and now they refuse to talk to me anymore because they think I put a curse on their marriage!

Love and Marriage: Here and Now

Here's a story about constantly shopping around for the perfect mate, one my guru told me a long time ago but that is unfortunately still relevant today.

Two men graduate college and get good jobs. One man gets married, has children and leads a wonderful life. The other man doesn't get married. The married man asks, "How come you never got married?"

The bachelor says, "I'm looking for a perfect woman for me. I just haven't found her yet."

After a couple of years he still hasn't found the perfect woman, so he moves to another town and continues his search. Decades go by. In the later years of his life, he returns to his hometown and he sees his old friend, still happily married and now surrounded by his children and grandchildren. The married man asks his friend, "So, you never found the perfect woman?"

The bachelor replies, "Yes, I finally did!"

The old friend says, "Great. Why don't you introduce her to us?"

"Because I'm not with her; I'm still not married" is the reply.

Perplexed, the married man says, "But I thought you said that when you found the perfect woman you would marry her."

"Yes, I did." The single man sighs. "But she said I was not the perfect man for her."

The moral of this story is what I've been telling you: Don't look for the perfect mate. Perfect yourself instead. Then just open your loving heart and allow other hearts to connect with yours. I pour these ideas about love and marriage into my students' brains and let them blend them like a strawberry milk shake. Once they taste that milk shake, it's the best they ever had!

For the last word on marriage, let's consider the sex part. You're paying attention now, am I right? Sex means what? A physical activity, a physical exchange? No. Real sex is soul-to-soul, mind-to-mind, body-to-body. Just body-to-body without the other parts is fake sex, bad sex—without real communication or fulfillment. You don't enjoy it; you become a machine. And even that machine breaks. After a few days, a few months, a few years, it doesn't work anymore. Then you look for somebody else; so does your partner.

Now let's say instead of breaking up and looking for different sex, you go to yoga class together. Now you have tremendous communication: body, mind and soul. This creates a beautiful, mutual understanding. Everything you do—cooking together, working together, driving someplace together, going on vacation together and yes, making love together—you enjoy a thousand times better. You are saying "Wow!" all over the place. Instead of one man making love to one woman, one yogi should make love to one yogini. Then instead of divorce, there will be a beautiful marriage—but only after the two partners have achieved happy marriages within themselves in their own bodies, minds and hearts.

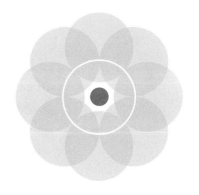

CHAPTER THIRTEEN

Second Stage, Part Two: Fulfilling Your Karma Yoga

THE SACRED DUTY WE ARE MEANT TO PERFORM IS PRESENT IN the entire span of your life, but this second segment, *Garahasthya*, is the most crucial time. If you were lucky enough to have a guru in your earlier years, he would have helped you to understand your destiny, and now you would begin to carry it out. If your Karma Yoga wasn't made clear to you before *Garahasthya*, now you will discover it, and begin pursuing your life's work.

259

If proper attention is paid and sincere effort is made, our Karma Yoga comes to define who we are.

As you now know, to perform your Karma Yoga—to do your job—first you will need good health. Without it, you cannot even show up for work. Second, you need your mind to be efficient and clear, so you can learn your work and excel at your job. Third, you must have the ability to set your mind to your task with perfect concentration. And as we've discussed, through your combined practice of Hatha and Raja Yoga, you can achieve these things. If you don't, your job will not get done. Listen, God hired you for your job and he doesn't have anyone sitting around waiting in case you don't do it.

How do you know what that job is? I told you that my guru could look at any child and see what that kid should become. He could read human beings from the inside out, and he was never wrong. He'd say, "Don't be a writer, be a scientist, a physicist. You can become another Einstein." This is a huge responsibility, and it requires special powers to see into people's souls, the same way a top-notch geologist can look at a pile of dirt and determine that there's gold buried under it. Then the geologist needs more people to get rid of the dirt, so that only the gold remains. Traditionally, the guru does both of those jobs: He discovers the hidden treasure in someone and then he digs down deep and hammers away all the useless material surrounding that gold. Without the skilled instruction of a master geologist, a teacher or guru, you might not ever find out what your special qualities are, or see what your gold can become. A human tragedy. But don't look so sad—there's a way to avoid this unhappy ending.

Karma Yoga: Here and Now

When you practice Hatha Yoga here in the Second Stage of your modern American life, you can actually become your own guru. *You* can discover where your *karma* lies, even without a guru's help, and how to best carry out your life's mission. After you've practiced with commitment for some time—when your body is no longer junked and your brain is not screw-loose—you open communication with the Spirit that has now awakened within you. Your true, best Self knows what your special gifts are, and how you can reach your ultimate potential, and *now* you can hear and understand your own inner wisdom, the voice of your true self.

Before you did yoga, you had a billion dollars in the bank—that's your buried gold—but you couldn't withdraw it because you didn't have the proper identification. Yoga is the access code, the PIN. Now through practice and self-observation you know what you are truly meant for and best at, you can see your path, and you can begin to realize the fulfillment of your Karma Yoga.

I think in some ways, having to serve as your own guru is actually better for you. As Americans, you prize independence so much—you're all about standing on your own two feet. From what I've seen, many people here would not be comfortable with humbling themselves the way a disciple must before his guru. If that total respect and devotion to the teacher is missing, then a guru can't teach you, anyway; he won't be able to help you with your mental, physical and Spiritual needs. So for most Americans, having a guru probably won't work. That's okay. Finding your own path could in itself be a part of your collective Karma Yoga—the American way.

What do you have to do to find your Karma Yoga here in the West, in the 21st century? Your first job in the Second Stage— all you need to focus on—is taking care of your body and mind. Do your yoga. You must become the janitor and the guard dog of your temple, protecting it and keeping it clean. Nothing from outside can come into the temple and harm it; otherwise *Atma*, the Spirit, will not be comfortable there. If a fire, flood or earthquake damages your home, you cannot live in it. In the same way, the Spirit cannot inhabit a broken home in which there's no water and no heat. In that case, there will be no unified Self and then you cannot see your path, much less travel it.

When you do honor your body temple and begin to achieve balance and union, all manner of cosmic doors and windows begin to open. Through them, you see to another level of consciousness. You let go of old wounds and all hatred. You begin to see the good in the universe, not just the bad, and you see the same goodness in yourself (after all, you are but a reflection of the universe).

When you reach this cosmic level you are reborn. You're not American or Indian, European or Arab, man or woman any longer. You're not Christian or Muslim, you're not black and you're not white. You are a human being. That is all, and at the same time, that is everything.

When you get to this higher level, you'll know what your life should be. If you have a good voice, now you can become the next Barbra Streisand. You showed talent in science? Now you can follow Einstein. Sometimes your path will be in the area in which you're already working and earning money to survive; sometimes it won't. But if you don't see your karmic path and accept the real duties of your life, you can end up in any old job, just doing it because somebody is paying you. No! That is not life. You are worth more than that.

I had one student who held a respectable job as an FBI officer for over 25 years. One morning, he woke up and said, "What am I doing?" He quit and became a yoga instructor. He doesn't charge any money—he goes around the world and he teaches for free, because he's able to do that.

Understand me, please: You don't have to quit what you're doing to follow your karmic path. Another student of mine is a very successful lawyer. He was involved in the Watergate hearings back in the 1970s. When he became my student (now he's my lawyer, too) he wasn't too happy about some of the work he did, the Mafia people and drug dealers he defended. Since he started yoga he now does cases for free, pro bono work, and he donates to charity. He didn't have to quit the law to become a better person.

In fact, he became an *even better* lawyer through yoga—he was more focused, with more willpower. He's more intuitive and has better stamina, too. Regardless of your profession, you will perform your job duties, as well as your karmic ones, better with yoga. You'll be a better husband or wife, and a better parent, too.

And as I described before, if you are not a successful person before you start your yoga, the practice and the *satsang* of happier, more successful people around you will lift you up. Often, I've seen people who've had a particular problem start helping people who have the same problem, such as a former drug addict becoming a substance abuse counselor. This is a beautiful *Karma*.

The risk for people who don't have a good foundation, don't do yoga, and don't understand that life is a four-stage progression, is that they can live their whole lives in the second quarter.

Family, work, work, family—soon they ask, Is that all there is? They stay trapped there, because they don't know they are supposed to move on. Because this is ultimately not very satisfying, they start to take wrong turns, make mistakes and develop bad habits. They're mixed up; they put curry powder on sushi, metaphorically speaking. Sushi tastes very good with wasabi—but curry will ruin it every time. You must learn to season your life with the proper choices, or you may suffer from karmic indigestion, my friend.

Often, the temptation is to stay in this second stage. If things appear to be going well, then that urge can be even stronger! We're so afraid of change, of possibly losing something, that we can't let go. But yoga tells us, Hey, it's time to move on. Time for the Third Stage of life.

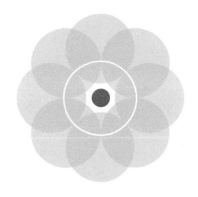

CHAPTER FOURTEEN

Third Stage: Service and Nonattachment

IN THE ANCIENT TRADITION, ALL THE COMPLEX EMOTIONAL, materialistic and sexual attachments you have just gone to so much trouble to form in the Second Stage are considered mere child's play. These attachments are just feelings we experience during what the holy men consider our formative years (even though you may be 55 to 70 years old at this point). You're done working to make a living and playing with your toys, and now in *Banaprasthya*, real life—spiritual life—begins. By consciously removing all of the attachments in your life, we were taught, you give yourself freedom to live.

Now older and wiser, no longer a boy with his toys, you say to yourself, "Enough is enough. I ate enough. I had enough sex, I drove enough cars, I wore enough nice clothes. I had enough property. I wanted them, but I don't need them anymore. I enjoyed myself all these years working hard, saving money, buying real estate, making investments, whatever. I realize now, though, when death seems so much nearer, that none of these things will prevent my inevitable death—and I can't take any of it with me. Absolutely nothing."

It's not just about renouncing *things*. Do you love your grandchildren? Good! Do you love your friends? Do you still love your wife? Good! Do you still look at a young woman or man and feel the deep stirrings of youthful attraction? Of course you do! Congratulations, you have successfully accumulated a wide range of emotional attachments and bound yourself to many different people.

Now leave them all. Walk away. Let them be.

Needless to say, this stage is acknowledged to be the hardest part of human life.

In India, you would go back to your guru's *ashram* or the place you were trained and teach for free, sharing your wisdom and experience with new generations. You would go alone. No more worries about money, sex and family, no more tension every day. You don't need money in the *ashram*—you perform your service there and they feed you.

In the Second Stage you took care of your children, but now they're old enough to take care of themselves. And you took care of your parents, like you are supposed to, but by now they may well be gone. If not, in India, they would have the rest of the extended family around them, and your mom and dad would realize that at this point you have different responsibilities to fulfill. They could go to an *ashram*, too, and get free accommodations, free food and free medicine.

Sexual attachment you don't have to worry about. That just goes with age, like a little dirt flushed from your fuel lines.

Third Stage: Here and Now

All this renouncing, going your way alone and doing without, sounds very severe, I know. It's a very tall order. I'm not about to tell every American to forget about their family and walk away— you won't do that, and there are no *ashrams* for you to go to, anyway. It's not practical, nor is it necessary to achieve Self-Realization. For our society, here and now, I emphasize two things:

1.   Detachment from material things

2.   Service, service, service

By now you should have made enough money, and saved enough, to have the bare necessities. That's all money is good for at this point; other than that, it gets you nowhere. In fact, it keeps you stuck in the Second Stage. Let go of your attachments to your stuff, your status and all the other aspects of materialism and then, a few years later, look back. You will see that nothing lasting has been left behind. You won't care how much money you had in the bank, how many girlfriends you had or how famous you were.

Instead you are doing service or social work. You become the guru, the teacher, the master or sensei. You dedicate yourself to serving the community, for free. Maybe you're a schoolteacher, a yoga teacher, a lifeguard; maybe you work in a soup kitchen or you drive people around who don't have a car. Don't fear that by deemphasizing your family and romantic attachments you will lose your humanity. It is your loved ones that have helped you to experience connection in a small circle—the next phase of life lets you widen your circumference. Now that the attachments to your loved ones are not as demanding and you are giving to others freely—to strangers, often—people actually become an even bigger part of your mind and Spirit. Of course, when you give of yourself like this, with an open hand, not demanding anything in return, you get back a thousand times more. I know about this because I'm a selfish man.

Why do I say that? I'll answer with another little story. The other day I'm at the gas station, filling up one of my cars, and a woman comes and asks me for a quarter; she says it's to feed her kitten. Maybe that's true, maybe not—what do I care? So I reach into my little bag and give her whatever money I have there; I think it was $5 or $7. This way I feed her kitten, but more important, I feed *my need* for emotional satisfaction. This is the highest-quality experience I can have, when I make another human being happy. When someone lets you do something for them, they don't need to thank you; you should thank *them* for making you feel good. As in: "Thank you so much for coming to my home to eat my food. You come again, I'll cook for you again, and again I'll be happy."

I am the one who gains here. I am the happiest person in the world because through my teaching I make so many thousands and thousands of people happy. That's the intelligence of the yogi, and that's why I say I am a selfish man.

What amazes me about our society, though, is that community service is not seen as the obligation or sacred duty of every man and woman—it's something the courts sentence criminals to! I see this all the time in the papers: "So-and-so was convicted and now he has to do this many hours of community service." Are you kidding me? What does that say about our culture? You shouldn't have to be *sentenced* to serve the community because you did something wrong. We should have the best people lining up to do this kind of giving! Service has nothing to do with incarceration; on the contrary, it means *liberation*.

When you reach your "retirement," let your money and possessions go out of your mind and try to maintain uncomplicated family relations, so you won't be distracted from your real job in this Third Stage: service to the community. Why not share all the wisdom and experience you have gained in your life? Help the younger generations learn from your mistakes and successes in order to better understand their own lives. Help them make a better world. You could teach yoga—I have helped many people become yoga teachers who were in their 50s, 60s and even their 70s. Why not? If enough readers of this book committed to teaching Hatha Yoga to our children just *one hour a week*, this country would be improved—blessed—immeasurably.

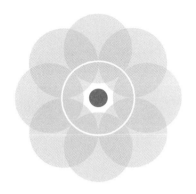

CHAPTER FIFTEEN

Fourth Stage: Higher Consciousness and the End of Life

AFTER THE THIRD STAGE OF BANAPRASTHYA, WHEN THE END of mortal life is approaching, the true yogi graduates to *Sannyas*. This is the ultimate holy path walked by those who choose the life of the ascetic. Like a Zen Buddhist monk, you find a place of great natural beauty, sit quietly, and spend the remainder of your life in constant meditation.

At this point you are so pure and your powers of concentration are so strong that you don't burn in fire, you don't sink in water, you don't freeze in the cold. You've learned to live entirely on *prana*, or cosmic energy. Should you care to, you can perform superhuman feats of strength or endurance. Maybe one day you even start to levitate.

If you are completely successful in releasing your fears and controlling your mind like Jesus, Buddha, Mohammed or Yogananda—all fully Realized human beings—you eventually become capable of conquering death. You are the one who decides one day to withdraw your Soul or Spirit voluntarily from the temple of your body in the act of *Mahasamahdi*. Your Spirit, *Atma*, reaches out to the Great Spirit, or Soul—*Mahatma*—and *Mahatma* reaches to *Paramahatma*, the Supreme Soul or God. You no longer have a material presence; only the Spirit lives on as part of the animating force of the Universe. This is the highest destiny achievable when one follows a yogic Spiritual path, and it happens in *Sannyas*.

Fourth Stage: Here and Now

Forget about it—this kind of enlightenment is not going to happen to very many people, here or in India, and for most of you I would say that attaining it is not even a proper goal. I just want you to understand the philosophical and Spiritual foundation of yoga and to appreciate also the supernatural power that is within us all. If some human beings can go this far, can reach this awesome level, just imagine what is available to you if you go just halfway!

What I do wish for you at this stage is to die with dignity. And before that to make sure your parents and grandparents die the same way. Here, I think America has a major problem. What I see happening to older people here horrifies me.

Go to any apartment building in any of our cities and what do you see? Older men and women with nothing but their TV and a bunch of cats and dogs to keep them company. Where are their sons and daughters? Where are their grandchildren? Or maybe these elderly people are warehoused in some old-age home run by strangers; they don't know these people from Adam. The message Western society is transmitting is that the elderly are useless or an unsavory burden, so let's dump them in the trash can. Even the language used to describe them diminishes them; they're called "little old ladies" and "dirty old men."

These are your parents and grandparents! They worked hard their entire lives, cooking food every day, raising children and giving them everything they could. Do they honestly deserve this kind of ending? This is not just a crime against them but against you, too, because you are a part of humanity. If you can't care for your own parents, then who can you ever really care for? Not yourself, certainly. The disease of indifference to our elders sickens all of our souls. We try to forget about it, but it's there.

In India the elderly are revered as treasures of wisdom and lore, as well as a connection to our past. My parents, grandparents and teachers have been the most important people in my life. It is my duty and honor to serve them. Even if you can't always save the day, you can still be there for them. Do you want to know how my father died? Our family and many other families were gathered around his bed (this was in India). People were chanting, incense was burning. My father had his head on my lap, one hand in my sister's hand, another hand holding my mom's hand, one foot touching my brother and another foot touching my sister-in-law. We were pouring water from the

Ganges River into his mouth, and the priest was chanting prayers.

That's the way everybody should die—peacefully, and in the company of the ones they love. Not one person saying to another, "Oh, Mr. Ford, have you seen Mrs. Smith? I haven't seen her for three or four days. Do you think she's all right?" Finally one of them calls 911, the police break down the door and it turns out Mrs. Smith has been dead for days but nobody even knew. We can't treat human beings—physical expressions of the divine—like that.

This is why—wish me luck—I want to build America's best active retirement community. The places that exist now cost way too much money. I'm not going to call my place an old-folks home, and the residents won't just sit around doing nothing all day, or playing cards. I'm going to make them busy 12 hours a day so these beautiful men and women will never think they're retired, or they're old. I'm going to do it, but I know it's not going to happen overnight.

Once again, this is a cultural problem. It's not that you don't love your parents; you just haven't seen a better way of caring for them demonstrated for you, so you can learn that this is how it's done. If you've never been taught the right way, you can end up doing things wrong and still think you're doing them right.

By striving for balance, for union—for yoga—you can create a marriage within you to heal the sickness that exists all around you. We can change ourselves, and we can therefore change our world.

Honor your parents and elders as you will wish to be honored when you reach the Fourth Stage of Life. Know that as you ride the wave-crest of youth, the trough of old age is before you. Once you've done that with your relatives, expand that circle of kindness to older people who aren't related to you, the Mrs. Smiths and Mr. Fords. Give love to get love back a thousandfold. You'll feel better: They'll feel better, everyone wins. When you serve them, you are ultimately serving yourself, and now you know in your heart that we are all equally deserving.

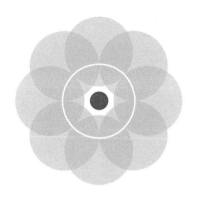

CHAPTER SIXTEEN

Your Time Is Now: Seeing the Good, Realizing the Self

As you implement your own version of the Four Stages of Life, the plan that suits your personality and your situation as a 21st-century American, continue practicing your Hatha Yoga. Under the supervision of a master mechanic, your body, mind and Spirit get more and more in tune. Along the way another miracle happens, as amazing in its own right as the transformation of your body and the gift of peace washing over your restless mind. Seeing this change occur in my students is one of the most cherished experiences I have as a teacher. It's so simple, but so powerful: You start to see the good things in life and forget about the bad.

I said that your practice will cause doors and windows to open and that through them, you will perceive things differently. Some call this the opening of your third eye, or Lord Shiva's eye, a cosmic energy center that sits invisibly between the eyebrows. Through these new ways of looking, you see only the good things in the universe. The two eyes you use most often have been taught to focus on the bad things first. Because of the negative power those attachments have, the force of negative attraction is nine times stronger than the attraction we feel to good things. But now with the third eye of consciousness, you can see the real nature of things and people, which is essentially good. Remember, God is love and God is within you. Always.

In my class and in the philosophy I teach, we don't criticize the bad—we appreciate the good, because the bad is limited, while the good is endless. Consider this: What's the worst thing that could happen to you? You die, so what. It's over and then you don't feel anything. Bad is insignificant and has an end.

When you experience bad things in your life, why feel bad? Things can only get better. So when things are bad, be happy. In India, we only get a little worried when things are going really, really good—because we know that in order to balance our lives, some bad stuff is probably just around the corner. But still, we enjoy the good.

Good is unlimited, infinite and abstract. Tell me: How much happiness can you have, how much peace, how much friendship, how much love? You can't tell me, because it's beyond human imagination. And until you practice yoga you will have no idea how much good you have *in you*. You've tapped into maybe 5 percent of your physical, mental and Spiritual power. You're sitting on a gold mine, or a diamond mine, or an oil field. But until you are able to dig beneath the surface, you'll never know, and you won't be able take advantage of that discovery. When you practice yoga and you begin to understand the goodness within you, you can see the world outside your own skin as good also.

It all starts from a perception inside. The "problems" we have exist only because you label certain things that way. You're making a judgment on a set of circumstances or events, and judging them as undesirable. What if you had the power to see the good in everything, and ignore the bad? What if you could take negative thoughts, emotions, words and actions, and transform them into their positive equivalent? Imagine all the extra energy and power you would possess. The simple truth is, *you can do this.* This is an important step on the path, an awakening or a kind of introduction to Self-Realization.

You know how easy it is to get angry over the simplest things. When someone confronts you with anger, don't you usually find yourself blindly falling into the same weakness, the same little trap they are in? It is much more challenging to derive laughter from rage or despair, and to act with faith, self-control, determination, concentration and patience instead of reacting out of blindness, weakness, fear and pain. The right way *is* the hard way. It is our responsibility to find the strength and discipline to do it.

Practicing Seeing the Good

These changes in your outlook—your beliefs about life—occur naturally when you practice Hatha Yoga, but you can also train yourself to see the positive. The next time you are stuck in traffic, for example—running late, feeling anxious and angry—

stop. Not the car; you're already bumper-to-bumper. Stop your negative thoughts. Ask yourself, Is there some good here that I am not seeing? How bad is my life really that I should let a few minutes' delay ruin everything?

One good trick is to imagine that you are watching yourself in the car, becoming furious. Then pull back, as if you are the cameraman and you are filming a movie—and congratulations, you're the star! Now you have a wider focus. What's really going on in this character's life? you ask yourself. Odds are, you are traveling to or from your very nice house, where you live with your beautiful family, in just one of the excellent vehicles you, your spouse and kids are lucky enough to own. Maybe you're nervous about being late because you want to do some work, to perform your job that many, many people in this country and around the world can only dream of holding.

I'm also betting you don't have a terminal disease that is going to kill you in the next 20 minutes. This traffic tie-up is not literally a life-or-death situation. Maybe it even gives you an opportunity to practice your *pranayama* breathing exercises for a little while, or to think about something that really deserves your attention but that you've been too busy—or too busy avoiding—to sit down and think about. Now you have time; if you're driving on the Pacific Coast Highway, you could have an hour or more! The key thing here is: Consider the big picture. See the good. Forget the bad.

This is the beginning of transformation. All lasting transformation requires the proper tools, from a mechanic's wrench to a mother's love. To reach Self-Realization we use the most sophisticated tools ever imagined: the human body and the human mind. And to integrate these master works of evolution with each other and with the Spirit, the very heart of God within us, we use the gift of the ancient sages, yoga. Through practicing yoga we can fully practice our humanity.

As human beings entering the 21st century, we have collectively reached the pinnacle of achievement in areas such as science, technology, art, commerce, athletics, music, economy, medicine and higher education. But for many, something is still missing. For some of us, it's simply good health; we lack the strength, flexibility and balance; the perfect marriage between heart and lungs; and the rejuvenating benefits of *pranayama* and *asana* in every part of our bodies to effectively fight off illness and disease. For others, what remains to be achieved is more mental and Spiritual than physical: the knowledge and ability to lead a happy life with true satisfaction. Again, balance is the missing element.

In reading this book you have educated yourself, and you have learned about the problems we face, why they exist, and their solutions. Now you must begin to *live* that solution through the practice of Hatha Yoga, for true knowledge and education is gained only through experience. All the philosophical ramblings and theological debate ever conceived put together can never substitute for the doing and feeling of individual experience. If your mind offers you any resistance, conjuring up excuses, all you have to do is remember the words of my guru, Bishnu Ghosh: *"It's never too late, it's never too bad, and you're never too old or too sick to start from scratch once again."*

We're each born with supernatural, cosmic power. It's within each and every human being, but by now you know the story: Having something doesn't mean anything if you don't know how to use it. You have to realize it, you have to process it, you have to achieve it. That's called life. This is the only way for human beings to break free from their self-imposed limitations and begin to understand that *there are no limitations*.

I don't know of a word in the English language that can adequately express the highest form of Spiritualism, but the idea that comes closest is *loyalty*. It's an echo of the Hindi word *prem*, which blends concepts of gratefulness, love, honor, respect and true friendship. I would best describe *prem* as finding the truth within your own heart and maintaining the courage to follow it. Staying loyal to the truth and the voice of God within us is the greatest Spiritual quality that you or I can ever possess. The science of yoga allows us to understand the language of this divine truth, and the practical means to uphold it. Stay true to your Self by demonstrating both English bulldog determination and Bengal tiger strength.

Can I, Bikram, do this for you? Is that my job? Not a chance. You must choose to change for your Self and by yourself. You must begin at the roots, and climb up to the highest branches. All I can do is show you the way. I am offering you my experience and the wisdom of the ancient tradition of Self-liberation that my guru taught me, and that a long line of yogis taught before that. So please don't give me any credit, but rather credit the accuracy of my memory. I'm giving you the message handed down to me because you need it, you deserve it, and lastly, because you paid for it.

You can do it. Tightly grip the steering wheel of your life, turn the master key in the ignition, shift into Drive and take back control of your life. It's so simple. Just open your eyes, open your heart and open your mind, and allow your Spirit to guide you on the road. Trust your Self to make the decisions that will lead you to peace, happiness and a true satisfaction in living. And once you do this, you can then help everybody else do it.

Though this book is a wake-up call and guide for all Americans, I must emphasize again that my message is universal. As I've said all along, the East isn't perfect either. What we need, and what I have begun with this book, is to merge the best of the West with the best of the East.

Too many people look outside of themselves for answers. That way, you are forever in the desert chasing a mirage, looking for a drop of water that you will never find. Look inside, and you will find that the answers are already there. You had a gallon of fresh water in your backpack the whole time! You were born with it; your mom gave it to you. Now that you know where it is, all you have to do is reach behind you and take it.

You don't have to worry about changing the world; just change yourself, and you will surely inspire the world to follow. The longest distance any of us ever has to travel to reach Self-Realization is 6 inches. Take your hand, right now, and touch yourself on the forehead with the tips of your fingers. That is where we all must start. Now, touch your fingertips to the center of your chest, right over your heart. That is our ultimate destination. Six inches lie between mind and heart, between ego and Spirit, between fear and love. Six inches is all that separates us from God. It is the true path to Self-Realization, and the way is lit by yoga.

Whether you were born in the East or the West is of no consequence. All roads eventually lead to the same place. By taking the best from both worlds, we can begin to heal the wounds of misunderstanding and separation that have caused us so much unnecessary suffering, make soul-to-soul connections, and make our world whole at last. The time has come for the union of a healthy body, a peaceful mind and the realized Soul within each one of us, and a reunion of all Earth's children and their Mother. The time has come for knocking down walls, for forgetting our fears and forgiving each other in the creation of a global civilization based upon the ideals of friendship, truth and love. The time has come for yoga. See you in class, my friend.

Index

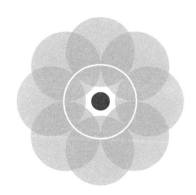